The
Thyroid
Diet

Also by Mary J Shomon

Living Well with Chronic Fatigue Syndrome and Fibromyalgia
What Your Doctor May Not Tell You About Parkinson's Disease
Living Well with Autoimmune Disease
Living Well with Hypothyroidism

The
Thyroid
Diet

Manage
your metabolism for
lasting weight loss

Mary J. Shomon

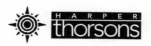

HARPER
thorsons

HarperThorsons
An Imprint of HarperCollins*Publishers*
77–85 Fulham Palace Road,
Hammersmith, London W6 8JB

The website address is: www.thorsonselement.com

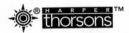

and *HarperThorsons* are trademarks of
HarperCollins*Publishers* Ltd

First published in the US by Harper*Resource* in 2004
First published in the UK by HarperThorsons in 2005

10 9 8 7 6 5 4 3 2 1

A catalogue record of this book
is available from the British Library

ISBN 0 00 721183 X

Printed and bound in Great Britain by
Creative Print & Design (Wales), Ebbw Vale

For Jeannie, my best friend,
through thin and thick and thin again

As long as the sky exists

And as long as there are sentient beings

May I remain to help

Relieve them of all their pain

– SHANTIDEVA'S PRAYER

Contents

PART 4: THE THYROID DIET

PART 5: MOVING FORWARD

APPENDICES

Acknowledgements

I'd like to thank my agent and friend, Carol Mann, who in her calm and steady way always manages to keep me headed in just the right direction. I am also extremely fortunate to have Sarah Durand at HarperCollins as my editor all these years. Her insightful editing and thoughtful approach pushes my work to levels I couldn't achieve without her guidance. I am so grateful to have these two talented and caring women in my life.

I am in awe of my husband, Jon Mathis, whose metabolism still makes me marvel, and I wish to thank him for his support, time, energy, love, and especially that pair of rose-colored glasses he's worn every time he has looked at me, even long before our wedding! Without him as my partner, my books would never become reality. And to both Jon and my daughter, Julia, who were patient and supportive (and did I say patient?) throughout the entire process of writing this book!

To my best friend, Jean-Marie Yamine, who is, as always, my sister, my Richelieu, my adviser, my personal pep squad, and the best brainstorming partner a writer could have.

And thanks to my dad, Dan, and my brother, Dan, for their support, and my mother, Pat, who even though she is gone, is with me always in heart and spirit.

Thanks also to my in-laws, Barbara and Russell Mathis, for their unfailing support, and for providing a safe and cozy haven for their son and granddaughter during my working weekends.

Many thanks to my dear aunt, Rita Kelleher, and my cousins, Ellen Blaze and Joan Kelleher, who are so supportive of me and my family.

I am indebted to Rosario Quintanilla and Elizabeth Mensah-Engmann for their many hours of caring for me and my family while I finished the book.

Many thanks to Jim McCauley, whose recipes and food ideas have truly changed the way I eat – buffalo burgers, who'd have thought? – and who has added so much to this book! And thanks to his partner, Edward Inderrieden, for his support of both Jim and me during the making of this book, and for willingly taste-testing all the recipes!

Kudos to Linda Souter and Paige Waehner, who were incredibly talented and diligent researchers and provided a great deal of assistance in putting together this book.

Continuing gratitude to Kate Lemmerman, MD, Bob Umlauf, PhD, and Silvia Treves, who keep me running smoothly, in both body and mind.

To all my dear friends on the Momfriends e-mail list for your support, cheers, camaraderie, and momvibes, during our more than 7-year daily cyberspace kaffeeklatsch!

To my unofficial news bureau, Rose Apter, Kim Carmichael-Cox, and health writer extraordinaire James Scheer, who regularly send me news reports, articles, and books that are right on target and always just what I need.

I must thank the many doctors, practitioners, and experts who provided information for the book, or who took time to brainstorm with me, shared their insights, or otherwise have contributed greatly to my thinking in the area of thyroid disease and nutrition. We are all fortunate to have these smart and caring people out there thinking about, researching, and caring for our health: Ken Blanchard, MD; David Brownstein, MD; Hyla Cass, MD; David Derry, MD; Udo Erasmus, PhD; Bruce Fife, ND, CN; Ted Friedman, MD; Ann Louise Gittleman, PhD; Donna Hurlock, MD; Dave Junno, PsyD; Stephen Langer, MD; Scott Levine, MD; Joseph Mercola, DO; Roby Mitchell, MD; Richard Podell, MD; Byron Richards, CCN; Marie Savard, MD; Karilee Halo Shames RN, PhD; Richard Shames, MD; Jacob Teitelbaum, MD; and Ken Woliner, MD.

Special thanks to Marisa Lavine and the Endocrine Society, Terry Dunkle of DietPower, Susan Burke of Ediets, Ric Rooney and Bart Hanks of PhysiqueTransformation, and Ray Faraee of Iherb for assistance and support.

And my heartfelt gratitude and commiseration to the thousands of people who have written to me to share their stories, pain, tears, laughter, joy, and sorrow as they go through this journey of thyroid disease and face the challenges of weight loss. I know exactly how you feel, and I can only hope that you find a glimmer of hope somewhere in this book, because you more than deserve hope, good health, happiness – and answers.

Introduction

I'm not afraid of storms,
for I'm learning to sail my ship.

— LOUISA MAY ALCOTT

Totie Fields once said, 'I've been on a diet for 2 weeks and all I've lost is 2 weeks.' If you're trying to lose weight, you may feel like Totie is talking about you. You may have tried diet after diet, joined Weight Watchers, tried herbal diet pills or read dozens of diet books that tell you to eat all protein, or cabbage soup or ice cream, or 1,000 or fewer calories per day, only to discover that you're not losing weight and might even be gaining it! That's what happened to me 10 years ago when I joined Weight Watchers, followed it to the letter, and gained 2 pounds a week while everyone else was losing weight.

Or you may never have had a weight problem, then all of a sudden, the pounds started piling on, seemingly defying all the laws of physics. If it takes 3,500 excess calories to gain a pound, how could you possibly have gained 10 or 20 pounds in 1 month? And yet you did. This is what happened to me at age 33 before my 1995 wedding. After going through my 20s as a slender size 10, I quickly started packing on weight – so much so that I bought a size 14 gown, and in the months before my wedding, I had to have my wedding dress let out two more sizes (is that a horrifying thing for a bride or what?). Even after I went on a reduced-calorie diet with daily exercise, I walked down the aisle as a size 18. After the honeymoon, the weight kept piling on.

Gena had a similar experience in her late 30s:

> I have a 20th school reunion coming up in my little hometown. I was always a perfect size, I played sport, and was a homecoming queen candidate. Sometime in my last year at secondary school, I woke up very sick one morning. The doctor told my mom that it was a thyroid infection. I took a lot of tests, got medication, and finally felt like my old self ... for maybe a year. What I didn't realize was the damage that was done to my thyroid gland would mess me up for the rest of my life. I gained weight from about 8 stones when I left school to about 14 stones at my top weight. And I *do not* eat any more than I used to; in fact, I'm eating much more healthily now. I'm depressed, because I've turned from a slender, healthy person into a person who just feels awful about her looks and is very embarrassed to go back to my hometown. If I could wear a sign that says 'I have a THYROID DISORDER' around my neck, maybe people wouldn't look at me and think, 'Look at that fat, lazy person ... she needs to push away from the table.'

Maybe you have been eating the same way as usual and getting the same level of physical activity as always, but you're wondering why this past six months you have managed to put on a pound a week.

In the midst of any of these situations, you may go to see your doctor, saying, 'I know something is really wrong with me.' And you may be sent home with one of the following:

A. **An antidepressant, because after all, depression makes you gain weight, so that must be it**
B. **A diet drug, because writing a prescription gives your doctor something useful and doctor-like to do**
C. **A shrug of the shoulders, along with one of those vague non-explanations like, 'Well, you are getting older – it's to be expected,' or 'It must be your hormones,' or 'It's normal after having a baby,' and so on**
D. **A condescending look, along with some serious medical advice along the lines of, 'Well, you must be eating too much and not getting enough exercise, so get off the couch and stop strapping on the feedbag!'**

Thanks, doc.

You know something is not right, and you know that you are not sitting around lazily stuffing your face with bonbons, but you don't get the feeling that the doctor believes you. And the sad fact is, he or she probably doesn't. One late 2003 study showed that not only GPs but even health professionals who specialize in treating obesity have negative stereotypes about people who are overweight, including associating them with being lazy, stupid and worthless. Most doctors – and the people around you, to an even greater extent – have an automatic anti-fat bias.

You *know* something is wrong – something is not normal – but who believes you?

I believe you.

Because while your doctor is busy assuming that you're too lazy to exercise and don't have enough willpower to stop eating, what he or she *isn't* doing is telling you that you could have a thyroid problem – a dysfunction in the small, butterfly-shaped gland in your neck that is crucial to your metabolism. While some narrow-minded doctors dismiss thyroid disease as just another lame excuse for being overweight, the reality is that for millions of overweight people, thyroid disease is a very real reason for weight problems. Learning about thyroid disease and its symptoms – beyond weight problems – and how to get diagnosed can be critical steps that address the underlying cause of your weight gain, help restore your hope and health, and allow a healthy diet and exercise to finally work the way they should!

Recent studies have conservatively estimated that as many as 20 million people have a thyroid problem, the majority of them undiagnosed. Some experts believe that the actual number is substantially higher and rapidly on the rise. At the same time, studies have shown that millions of us are overweight or obese.

This brings up a critical connection: some people struggling with a weight problem are facing even more of an uphill battle than everyone else, because they are dealing with an underlying thyroid condition that is both undiagnosed and untreated. One study found that as many as 40 per cent of overweight people had evidence of a dysfunctional thyroid.

I went to the doctor a number of times complaining about a variety of symptoms such as:

- Unexpected weight gain, despite diet and exercise
- Fatigue and exhaustion
- More hair loss than usual
- Moodiness
- Muscle and joint pains and aches
- Loss of sex drive

My doctor took a 'wait-and-see' approach for a few months, but then she put together the symptoms and decided she should test my thyroid. I was surprised when she called to say that I was hypothyroid. I didn't even know what a thyroid was. Sure, I'd heard overweight people laughingly referred to as having glandular problems, and I had an aunt who'd had a goitre once, but that was the extent of my knowledge about the master gland of metabolism.

My doctor put me on thyroid hormone replacement therapy. Blissfully ignorant, I assumed that all the symptoms, particularly the pounds, would disappear as quickly as they had appeared now that I was getting my thyroid back in order.

Surprise! Not so ...

Sure, as we tweaked my medicine and dosages, I felt better in some ways – less exhausted, not so moody and achy – but except for a few pounds, the weight didn't budge. In my 20s, before my thyroid apparently started to go awry, losing weight was simple. I just cut out a bag of crisps with lunch a few times a week and switched to a diet soda instead of regular, and within a few weeks the extra pounds would be gone.

But nothing I was doing in the beginning moved the scales an ounce. This wasn't going to be so easy. So I set out on a mission. To discover how best to optimize my thyroid treatment. To learn what and how much I could and couldn't eat in order to lose weight. To find out whether I needed to exercise, what type of exercise, and how much. To learn how to get back on track when my weight-loss efforts got stalled or even derailed.

Along the way, I turned my own struggle to find the answers into a new role as a patient advocate for others with thyroid and autoimmune diseases. In 1997, I started several websites and newsletters that focus on thyroid disease and the issues that patients face. They have become the most popular patient-oriented thyroid websites on the Internet. My first book, *Living Well with Hypothyroidism*, has gone on to more than 20 printings and a second edition. And my *Thyroid Diet Success Guide*, a simple 40-page summary of weight-loss tips that was the inspiration for this book, has inspired thousands of thyroid patients to lose weight successfully. Throughout it all have been the thousands of letters each month from people all around the world describing their symptoms, asking if they could have a thyroid problem, and discussing their inexplicable frustration with their weight gain and their misery over not feeling well. Thyroid patients asking why they have not lost weight, despite rigorous diets and exercise programmes. People who said they cried as they wrote their e-mails that describe how being overweight makes them feel ugly, old, worthless and unattractive, and nothing has worked in their attempts to get the weight off.

Along the way, I've been on my own journey, and it's taken me almost 10 years to figure out what I needed to know. And now I'm sharing it with you in *The Thyroid Diet*.

You don't want to be overweight. I know there is a percentage of people who are overweight who feel comfortable with themselves and don't have any body image issues, and more power to them. But I'm not one of them, and if you're reading this book, neither are you.

When I've been overweight, I haven't been proud to be fat. Like doctors and most of the public, I see being overweight as a failing, as a sign that I'm *less*. I don't need to be model-thin. I just want to feel and look normal, healthy and attractive. And most likely, so do you.

Let's face it: In addition to the psychosocial burden – basically, suffering emotionally or mental health-wise because of the self-esteem and depression issues related to being overweight – there is also an increased risk of many serious health conditions, including:

- Insulin resistance
- Diabetes
- High blood pressure
- High cholesterol
- Cardiovascular disease/heart disease
- Stroke
- Asthma
- Arthritis/degenerative joint disease
- Gallbladder disease

- Sleep apnoea
- Fatigue
- Complications of pregnancy
- Menstrual irregularities
- Stress incontinence

Being overweight or obese is also a risk factor for various cancers. A 16-year study by the American Cancer Society found that deaths from a wide variety of cancers – including those of the breast, endometrium, colon, rectum, oesophagus, pancreas, kidney, gallbladder, ovary, cervix, liver and prostate, as well as multiple myeloma and non-Hodgkin's lymphoma – are linked to excess weight and obesity. Only a few cancers – lung cancer, bladder cancer, brain cancer and melanoma – were found to have no link to excess weight. That's certainly enough incentive to lose weight.

But we have to get off the weight-loss run-around. If you read the newspapers and women's magazine articles, watch middle-of-the-night infomercials, view television interviews and talk to the staff at supplement stores, you'll hear from 'experts' galore, and every one of them has the one key to weight-loss success. The key is:

Detoxing the liver
Regulating insulin
Avoiding carbohydrates
Staying away from the wrong carbohydrates
Restricting calories
Not eating enough calories
Combining the right foods
Eating good fats
Following a low-fat diet
Eating raw foods
Juicing
Eating vegetarian
Following a high-protein diet
Grazing all day
Eating Mediterranean style
Exercising
Taking supplements

Taking weight-loss drugs

Eating cabbage soup

Following a liquid diet

Having surgery

Managing your mind and emotions

Regulating brain chemistry

'Figuring out why being fat is working for you'

(That last one is courtesy of Dr Phil.)

Blah blah blah!

The bottom line: *There is no single answer.* What works for *you* is the right answer. And that may be one of the above things, or far more likely, a combination of approaches.

Many, many people in Britain are overweight. And let's face it, while some have an underlying thyroid problem, some haven't. Yet most overweight people find it very hard to lose weight, because dropping pounds and keeping them off is very difficult. It's even tougher with a thyroid condition.

You're not lazy or lacking willpower. Your weight problem is most likely not an emotional issue that can be shouted and bullied out of you by a television personality. You're probably not downing an entire box of donuts every night when no one else is watching. Your eating habits are probably not very different from those of your friends or family members who are at a normal weight. Your body may truly refuse to lose weight on rabbit food, Weight Watchers or the Atkins diet.

Your problem is that your body doesn't work the way it's supposed to. A challenge that is already hard for most people may be even harder for you. This is the most difficult point to get past – to accept that fundamentally your thyroid condition may make weight loss an unfair fight, especially in the beginning and perhaps for ever. What you suspect about your body is probably true. You may gain weight more easily than others, and you probably won't lose weight as quickly as others.

In fact, if you are hypothyroid, your metabolism becomes so efficient at storing every calorie that even the most rigorous diet and exercise programmes may not work. Your friend or spouse could go on the same diet as you, lose a pound or two a week, and you might stay the same or even gain weight. *It's not fair!*

CAN WE SHOUT THAT TOGETHER? IT'S NOT FAIR!!!

OK, since we've established that it's not fair, it's time to move on. That's life – I've got a thyroid problem, you've got a thyroid problem, and it's not likely to go away. This is something we'll probably both live with for the rest of our lives. The question is: Are we going to live *well* with it, or is it going to define us and make us miserable? Is it going to stop us from feeling good about ourselves, fitting into clothes we like, feeling sexy, exercising or playing sports, having energy for work, family and children?

I made a decision that it wasn't going to stop me, and I hope you join me in that decision. That is where *The Thyroid Diet* comes in. I'm not going to tell you that you'll find any magic weight-loss secrets in this book. No miracle pill that will make the pounds melt away, or food that will allow you to eat all you want and lose weight overnight. I wish I had that to give you. (I wish I had it myself!)

But for those of you whose weight challenges are due to a thyroid condition that you don't yet know you have, what you will find in *The Thyroid Diet* are clear guidelines and straightforward information about thyroid disease that will help you find out more and get that diagnosis! *The Thyroid Diet*, in a simple, understandable way, offers you the support, encouragement and information you need to pursue the right diagnosis and treatment with your doctor. That's no easy task in today's environment of rigid diagnostic criteria and 10-minute managed-care visits.

The best news so far? Excitingly, for some of you, just getting treatment for your previously undiagnosed thyroid problem will be all that you need to return to a healthy weight, without a rigorous change in your diet and exercise!

However, for the majority of thyroid patients, treatment alone doesn't seem to resolve weight problems. Losing weight involves optimizing the thyroid treatment programme, because you may not be able to lose weight until you are on the right brand, mix and dosage of thyroid medicine. Simply switching brands, or adding an additional drug, or slightly changing dosages may be the minor adjustment that restores your metabolism to normal and allows you to lose weight. Again, *The Thyroid Diet* will help, as we explore the brands, mixtures and dosage options that may be right for you, along with other lifestyle issues and supplements to help optimize your thyroid treatment.

But despite optimal thyroid treatment, you may still struggle. At that point, other approaches become central to losing weight, including ensuring that your metabolism works as best it can, resolving underlying nutritional deficiencies, treating depression and correcting brain chemistry imbalances, reducing stress, combating insulin resistance, treating food allergies and sensitivities, and exercising. *The Thyroid Diet* will help you understand these factors. Herbs and supplements, stress-reduction techniques, prescription weight-loss drugs, ways to deal with food sensitivities, exercise guidelines and even innovative approaches like mesotherapy might help you get on track.

I've interviewed hundreds of doctors, extensively reviewed the latest research on thyroid disease, metabolism, weight loss and nutrition, and talked to thousands of thyroid patients over the past seven years. I've culled through this vast sea of information to share with you the best tips, ideas, theories and recommendations.

Perhaps most important are the actual eating plans. In *The Thyroid Diet* you'll find several different approaches, ranging from a less structured programme to options for those who are calorie and carbohydrate sensitive, to a more structured approach. You'll find food lists and a host of innovative suggestions that can help you get to a healthier weight. I know you'll find ideas that will work for you.

We even have a set of delicious and healthy gourmet recipes – consider them incentive! – from pioneering chef Jim McCauley, who as a food connoisseur and recently diagnosed diabetes sufferer has made it his mission to transform mundane healthy eating into a satisfying gourmet experience! You'll also find that the Appendices include information on books, websites, tools, support groups and experts who can help.

Isn't it time you mastered your master gland of metabolism? Let's get started!

PART 1

The Thyroid Connection

CHAPTER 1

Could You Have an Undiagnosed Thyroid Condition?

> Knowledge is of two kinds: we know a
> subject ourselves, or we know where we
> can find information about it.
>
> – SAMUEL JOHNSON

The thyroid is a small bowtie- or butterfly-shaped gland located in your neck around the windpipe, behind and below your Adam's apple area. The thyroid produces several hormones, but two are absolutely essential: triiodothyronine (T3) and thyroxine (T4). These hormones help oxygen get into your cells and are critical to your body's ability to produce energy. This role in delivering oxygen and energy makes your thyroid the master gland of metabolism.

The thyroid has the only cells in the body capable of absorbing iodine. It takes in the iodine obtained through food, iodized salt or supplements and combines that iodine with the amino acid tyrosine. The thyroid then converts the iodine/tyrosine combination into the hormones T3 and T4. The '3' and '4' refer to the number of iodine molecules in each thyroid hormone molecule.

Of all the hormones produced by your thyroid when it is functioning properly, approximately 80 per cent will be T4 and 20 per cent will be T3. Of the two, T3 is the biologically active hormone – the one that actually has an effect at the cellular level. So while the thyroid produces some T3, the rest of the T3 needed by the body is actually formed when the body converts T4 to T3. Once released by the thyroid, the T3 and T4 travel through the bloodstream. The purpose is to help cells convert oxygen and calories into energy to serve as the basic fuel of your metabolism.

As mentioned, the thyroid produces some T3. But the rest of the T3 needed by the body is actually formed from the mostly inactive T4 by a process sometimes referred to as T4-to-T3 conversion. This conversion can take place in the thyroid, the liver, the brain and in other organs and tissues.

As T3 circulates through your bloodstream, it attaches to and enters your cells via receptor sites on the membrane of the cells. Once inside the cells, T3 increases cell metabolic rate, including body temperature, and stimulates the cells to produce a number of different hormones, enzymes, neurotransmitters and muscle tissue. T3 also helps your cells use oxygen and release carbon dioxide, which helps smooth metabolic function.

So how does the thyroid know how much T4 and T3 to produce? The release of hormones from the thyroid is part of a feedback process. The hypothalamus, a part of the brain, emits thyrotropin-releasing hormone (TRH). The release of TRH tells your pituitary gland to in turn produce thyroid-stimulating hormone (TSH). This TSH that circulates in your bloodstream is the messenger that tells your thyroid to make the thyroid hormones T4 and T3, sending them into your bloodstream. When there is enough thyroid hormone, the pituitary makes *less* TSH, which is a signal to the thyroid that it can slow down hormone production. It's a smoothly functioning system when it *works properly*. When something interferes with the system and the feedback process doesn't work, thyroid problems can develop.

PREVALENCE

Experts estimate that over half of all thyroid sufferers are undiagnosed. The majority of people with thyroid conditions have Hashimoto's disease, an autoimmune condition that causes hypothyroidism – an underactive thyroid. Thyroid disease is among the most common autoimmune conditions in the UK.

Women are seven times more likely than men to develop thyroid problems. Women face as much as a one-in-five chance of developing a thyroid problem during their lifetime. The risk of thyroid disease increases with age; by age 74, the 16 per cent prevalence of subclinical hypothyroidism in men is nearly as high as the 21 per cent rate seen in women.

Thyroid cancer is among the fastest-growing cancers. The incidence has increased 20 per cent since the late 1990s; experts believe this is due to increased radiation exposure from, for example, x-rays.

Thyroid problems are also common in many other countries, particularly areas covered at one time by glaciers, where iodine is not present in the soil and in foods. In many of these countries, an enlarged thyroid, known as goitre, is seen in as many as one in five people and is usually due to iodine deficiency. Around the world, an estimated 8 per cent of the population has goitre, most commonly women. Thyroid problems, including autoimmune thyroid disease and thyroid cancer, are more prevalent in the areas around and downwind of the 1986 Chernobyl nuclear accident.

OVERVIEW OF CONDITIONS

The main conditions that can occur with the thyroid include:

- **hypothyroidism – when the thyroid is underactive and isn't producing sufficient thyroid hormone**
- **hyperthyroidism – when the thyroid is overactive and is producing too much thyroid hormone**
- **goitre – when the thyroid becomes enlarged, due to hypothyroidism or hyperthyroidism**
- **nodules – when lumps, usually benign, grow in the thyroid, sometimes causing it to become hypothyroid or hyperthyroid**
- **thyroid cancer – when lumps or nodules in the thyroid are malignant**
- **postpartum thyroiditis – when the thyroid is temporarily inflamed, in addition to hypothyroidism or hyperthyroidism triggered after pregnancy**

Causes and Risk Factors

The most common causes of thyroid conditions are autoimmune diseases, notably Hashimoto's thyroiditis and Graves' disease, where the body's immune defences inappropriately target the thyroid as an invader.

Hashimoto's disease may cause periods of hyperthyroidism, followed by permanent hypothyroidism after the immune system destroys the gland's ability to produce thyroid hormone. Graves' disease typically causes an overproduction of thyroid hormone which can become life-threatening if not treated. If you have Graves' disease, you'll most likely receive anti-thyroid drugs, radioactive iodine, or surgery that will partially or entirely disable the thyroid's ability to produce thyroid hormone. Most people will become hypothyroid after treatment for Graves' disease.

The risk of developing thyroid disease is greatest if:

- you or a family member has a history of thyroid problems
- you or a family member has a history of autoimmune disease (e.g. rheumatoid arthritis, psoriasis, vitiligo, multiple sclerosis, lupus, or other conditions)
- you are or were a smoker
- you have had a stomach infection or food poisoning in the past, especially if diagnosed as the food-borne bacteria *Yersinia enterocolitica* infection
- you have allergies or a sensitivity to gluten, or have been diagnosed with coeliac disease
- you've been exposed to radiation, by living near or downwind from a nuclear plant, or through particular medical treatments (e.g. treatment for Hodgkin's disease, nasal radium therapy, radiation to tonsils and neck area), or were nearby or downwind of the Chernobyl nuclear disaster in 1986
- you've been treated with lithium or amiodarone
- you have been taking supplemental iodine, kelp, bladder wrack and/or bugleweed
- you live in an area (e.g. the Midwestern 'Goitre Belt' in the US) where there is low iodine in the soil and you have cut down on the iodized salt in your diet, leaving you iodine deficient
- you've been exposed to certain chemicals (e.g. perchlorate) via your water, food or employment
- you've been excessively exposed to metals such as mercury and toxins such as environmental oestrogens and pesticides
- you use fluoridated water and have dental fluoride treatments
- you are a heavy consumer of soy products, especially soy powders or soy-based supplements

- you eat a substantial quantity of raw 'goitrogenic' foods such as Brussels sprouts, rutabaga, turnips, kohlrabi, radishes, cauliflower, African cassava, millet, babassu (a palm-tree coconut fruit popular in Brazil and Africa), cabbage and kale
- you are over 60
- you are female
- you are in a period of hormonal variance such as the perimenopause, menopause, pregnancy, or postpartum
- you have had serious trauma to the neck such as whiplash from a car accident or a broken neck
- you currently have or have in the past been diagnosed with the following diseases or conditions, known to occur more frequently in people with thyroid disease:
  - Other pituitary or endocrine disease (e.g. diabetes, a pituitary tumour, polycystic ovary syndrome [PCOS], endometriosis, premature menopause)
  - Chronic fatigue syndrome/ME
  - Fibromyalgia
  - Carpal tunnel syndrome/tendonitis/plantar fasciitis
  - Mitral valve prolapse syndrome (MVPS)
  - Epstein-Barr virus (EBV)
  - Glandular fever/Mononucleosis
  - Depression
  - Infertility or recurrent miscarriage
  - Coeliac disease/gluten intolerance

Various thyroid disease risk factors, along with a comprehensive list of symptoms, are featured in the checklist at the end of this chapter.

HYPOTHYROIDISM

The most common thyroid condition is hypothyroidism. If you have hypothyroidism, your thyroid fails to produce sufficient levels of the thyroid hormones needed by your body. This slows down a variety of bodily functions, as well as your metabolism. The risk of developing hypothyroidism is greatest if:

- an autoimmune disease (Hashimoto's disease) has caused your immune system to attack your thyroid, making it unable to produce sufficient hormone amounts
- you've had radioactive iodine (RAI) treatment for your overactive thyroid, which has made all or part of your thyroid unable to produce hormone
- you have a goitre or thyroid nodule(s) that is interfering with your gland's ability to produce hormone
- you've had surgery for goitre, nodules, Hashimoto's disease, or cancer and all or part of your thyroid has been removed.
- you've been hypothyroid since birth. A small percentage of people experience this condition, known as congenital hypothyroidism, which results from a missing or malformed thyroid gland.

Ultimately, however your thyroid problem started, if your thyroid is now unable to produce sufficient thyroid hormone, or if you haven't got a thyroid at all, you are considered hypothyroid.

Symptoms

You may be hypothyroid if:

- you are extremely exhausted and fatigued
- you feel depressed, moody and/or sad
- you're sensitive to cold and you have cold hands and/or feet
- you're experiencing inappropriate weight gain, or having difficulty losing weight, despite changes in diet and exercise
- your hair is dry, tangled and/or coarse
- you've lost hair, maybe even from the outer part of the eyebrows
- you have dry and/or brittle nails
- you're feeling muscle and joint pains and aches
- you have carpal tunnel syndrome or tendonitis in the arms and legs
- your soles of your feet are painful, a condition known as *plantar fasciitis*
- your face, eyes, arms or legs are abnormally swollen or puffy
- you have an abnormally low sex drive
- you have unexplained infertility, or recurrent miscarriages with no obvious explanation

- your menstrual period is heavier than normal, or your period is longer than it used to be or comes more frequently
- you feel like your thinking is fuzzy (e.g. difficulty concentrating, difficulty remembering)
- you're constipated
- you have a full or sensitive feeling in the neck
- your voice is raspy or hoarse
- you have periodic heart palpitations
- your total cholesterol and 'bad' (LDL) cholesterol levels are high and may not even respond to diet or medication
- your allergies have got worse and you experience symptoms such as itching, prickly hot skin, rashes and hives (urticaria)
- you regularly have infections, including yeast infections, oral fungus, thrush or sinus infections
- you feel shortness of breath, sometimes a difficulty drawing a full breath, or a need to yawn

Dana described how she determined that she needed to be tested for hypothyroidism:

> I have a Master's degree in nutrition and had worked for about eight years in health care at the time as a clinical dietician. The crunch for me came when I put a woman on a weight-loss diet. I asked her to eat about 1,800 calories per day and try to do 10 minutes on the treadmill daily. Meanwhile, I was doing 1½ hours of step aerobics daily and riding my bike to and from work and eating a strict (and I mean strict!) 1,200-calorie-a-day diet. She lost 8 pounds in a week, while I *gained* 2!

Dana's doctor was astute enough to suspect hypothyroidism straight away and she was diagnosed and able to get on a treatment programme.

Diagnosis

One possible sign of thyroid abnormality is a low basal body temperature. Some practitioners even believe that it can be indicative of hypothyroidism. Use a basal thermometer or mercury thermometer and take your temperature upon awakening before getting out of bed and moving around. Typically, basal body temperatures lower than 97.8 to 98.2 degrees Fahrenheit (36.5 to 36.7 degrees C) are thought to indicate hypothyroidism. This self-testing method was popularized by the late Dr Broda Barnes. This test is not considered conclusive by many practitioners and does not definitively diagnose or rule out thyroid abnormalities.

To diagnose or rule out hypothyroidism, conventional doctors will typically start with a blood test that measures thyroid-stimulating hormone (TSH). Other blood tests that may be done to help diagnose hypothyroidism include:

- total T4 (total thyroxine) – a low level along with an elevated TSH may indicate hypothyroidism
- free T4 (free thyroxine) – a low level along with an elevated TSH may indicate hypothyroidism
- total T3 – a low level along with an elevated TSH may indicate hypothyroidism
- free T3 – a low level along with an elevated TSH may indicate hypothyroidism
- anti-thyroid antibodies (thyroglobulin and microsomal) – the positive presence of antibodies usually indicates autoimmunity and possibly Hashimoto's thyroiditis or Graves' disease
- anti-thyroid peroxidase (anti-TPO) antibodies – the presence of antibodies usually indicates auto-immunity and possibly Hashimoto's thyroiditis or Graves' disease

Hashimoto's thyroiditis is the most common cause of hypothyroidism. The characteristic Hashimoto's thyroiditis patient has high TSH values and usually low T3 and T4 thyroid hormone levels. However, the greatest distinguishing feature for Hashimoto's is a high concentration of thyroid auto-antibodies – anti-TPO antibodies in particular. Some patients have elevations in antibody levels for months or even years before elevation of the TSH level.

If you would like to start with self-testing, you can do a home TSH test. A company called Biosafe received US Food & Drug Administration (FDA) approval for an accurate, affordable home TSH test. Biosafe's test kit requires an almost painless finger prick using a special finger lancet. All you need is a couple of drops of blood, which you put into a collection device and send to Biosafe's labs for analysis. Results are mailed back to you quickly. For information or to order a test, visit the website http://www.goodmetabolism.com.

Treating Hypothyroidism

Conventional treatment for hypothyroidism is with prescription thyroid hormone replacement drugs, which are almost always taken daily. Options are summarized in the following table.

THYROID HORMONE REPLACEMENT DRUGS

Name	Description
Synthetic T4	The most common treatment, provides synthetic version of one hormone, T4. Different brands may have different fillers, dyes and potential allergens.
Synthetic T3	Drug that is often given with T4
Synthetic T4 + T3	A combination synthetic drug
Time-released, compounded T3	Currently available only from compounding pharmacies
Natural, desiccated thyroid	Derived from thyroid gland of pigs, includes T4, T3 and other thyroid hormones including T1 and T2.

Most commonly, a T4 drug is prescribed, as this is considered the 'standard' treatment for hypothyroidism. Research and clinical practice by many thyroid experts has shown that some patients feel better with the addition of T3, so increasing numbers of practitioners are prescribing T4 plus T3 or, less commonly, T4 plus compounded T3. Another option is a synthetic T4 plus T3 combination drug, which is a safe and effective option for some patients.

From the early 1900s to the 1950s, the only form of thyroid-replacement drug available was natural, desiccated thyroid. The drug fell out of favour with some endocrinologists, as synthetic T4 was marketed as a better, more modern option for thyroid treatment in the second half of the 20th century. Marketing efforts aside, since the 1990s, natural, desiccated thyroid has been enjoying a resurgence in popularity with some patients and practitioners. Derived from the desiccated thyroid gland of pigs, the drug contains natural forms of numerous thyroid hormones and nutrients typically found in a real thyroid gland, and some patients report improvement in symptoms using natural thyroid versus the synthetic options.

A new thyroid drug is in development. The drug includes both T4 and T3 but will deliver the thyroid hormone in a slow-release pill form. It is meant to simulate the way the body actually releases thyroid hormone, avoiding the ups and downs in energy, pulse/heart rate and side-effects some patients experience from their thyroid drugs. Such a drug could be an improvement on the current thyroid hormone replacement treatments currently available.

In the case of Hashimoto's disease, if you test positive for antibodies but do not have an elevated TSH level, many practitioners will not treat you until your TSH level rises above the normal range. Other practitioners, however, treat with thyroid-replacement drugs to prevent worsening of autoimmune thyroid disease. This practice of treating patients who have Hashimoto's thyroiditis but normal-range TSH levels is supported by a study reported in the March 2001 issue of the journal *Thyroid*. In this study, German researchers reported that use of thyroid-replacement drugs for cases of autoimmune Hashimoto's disease where TSH had not yet elevated beyond normal range could reduce the incidence and degree of autoimmune disease progression. Scientists speculated that it might even be able to stop the progression of Hashimoto's disease or prevent hypothyroidism.

In Hashimoto's disease, around 10 per cent of patients actually have a spontaneous remission, typically from 4 to 8 years after starting thyroid hormone replacement. This remission is also associated with the disappearance of antibodies.

HYPERTHYROIDISM

Hyperthyroidism occurs when the thyroid is overactive, producing more thyroid hormone than is necessary. Just as hypothyroidism slows down the body's functioning, hyperthyroidism speeds it up, causing accelerated heart rate, high blood pressure and other concerns. Hyperthyroidism may be caused by:

- an autoimmune disease (Graves' disease) that has caused the immune system to attack the thyroid. Auto-antibodies bind to the thyroid gland and cause the thyroid to overproduce thyroid hormone.
- autoimmune Hashimoto's disease, a characteristic of which is a short spurt of overactivity before the thyroid shifts into underactivity
- a goitre, nodule, or nodules that have caused the thyroid to inappropriately produce too much thyroid hormone
- excessive exposure to iodine
- thyroiditis, an inflammation of the thyroid that makes the thyroid overactive
- being hypothyroid and taking too much thyroid medication.

Symptoms

Hyperthyroid patients often have an enlarged thyroid, which can be felt by a doctor upon examination. You may be hyperthyroid if:

- you're rapidly losing weight, or you are eating more and not gaining weight
- you're having a hard time falling asleep or staying asleep
- you're suffering from anxiety, irritability, nervousness or even panic attacks
- you're finding it difficult to concentrate
- you're having palpitations, or your pulse and heartbeat are rapid and blood pressure is elevated
- you're sweating more than usual, feeling hot when others are not
- you have tremors in your hands
- you're suffering from diarrhoea
- you feel tired

- your skin is dry, or you may even have a thickening of the skin on the shin area of your legs
- your periods have stopped or are very light and infrequent
- you're having muscle pain and weakness, especially in the upper arms and thighs
- you're having eye problems, such as double vision or scratchy eyes, or you notice that your eyes are bulging or more whites are showing than usual
- you're having trouble getting pregnant
- your hair has become fine and brittle
- your behaviour is erratic.

Diagnosis

A diagnosis is usually made by a thyroid-stimulating hormone (TSH) test. Anything lower than the 0.3 to 0.5 range would likely be diagnosed as hyperthyroid.

Other blood tests that may be done to help diagnose hyperthyroidism include:

- total T4 (total thyroxine) – a high level along with a low TSH may indicate hyperthyroidism
- free T4 (free thyroxine) – a high level along with a low TSH may indicate hyperthyroidism
- total T3 – a high level along with a low TSH may indicate hyperthyroidism
- free T3 – a high level along with a low TSH may indicate hyperthyroidism.

Additionally, the thyroid-stimulating antibodies (TSAb) or thyroid-stimulating immunoglobulin (TSI) in your blood may also be measured to diagnose Graves' disease, the autoimmune condition that frequently causes hyperthyroidism.

A radioactive picture of the thyroid that is made by ingesting radioactive iodine by mouth may also be taken to see if the thyroid gland is overactive. This overactivity is a hallmark of Graves' disease. (Note: Because radioactivity can potentially damage the unborn or breast-feeding infant's thyroid gland, this procedure is not done if you are pregnant or breast-feeding.)

Treating Hyperthyroidism

Regardless of the method of treatment eventually used, as a first course of action a doctor may initially recommend that you take a beta-adrenergic blocking drug – also known as a beta blocker – such as atenolol (Tenormin), nadolol (Corgard), metoprolol (Lopresor), or propranolol (Inderal) to block the action of circulating thyroid hormone in your tissue, slow your heart rate and reduce nervousness. These drugs can be useful in rapidly reducing potentially dangerous symptoms until treatment has taken effect.

When the disease is mild, or occurs in children or young adults, or needs to be promptly controlled (as with elderly patients whose heart disease puts them at risk from the increased heart rate associated with Graves' disease), the first main treatment approach is often a course of anti-thyroid drugs. These drugs make it more difficult for your thyroid to use the iodine it needs to produce thyroid hormone, resulting in a decrease in thyroid hormone production.

Anti-thyroid drugs work for about 20 to 30 per cent of patients. In some patients, anti-thyroid drug treatment for 12 to 18 months will result in prolonged remission of the disease, particularly if the disease is relatively mild when treatment is begun. These drugs can offer as much as a 40 per cent chance of remission in some patients. This is another reason to see your doctor early if you suspect you have the disease.

In about 5 per cent of cases, anti-thyroid drugs cause allergic reactions such as skin rashes, hives and sometimes fever and joint pains. A rarer and even more serious potential side-effect is a decrease in the white blood cells that are part of the immune system, thereby resulting in a decrease in resistance to infection. In very rare cases, these cells may disappear entirely (a condition called *agranulocytosis*), which can be potentially fatal if there is a serious infection.

If you experience an infection while taking these drugs, call your doctor immediately. The doctor will likely tell you to stop taking the drug straight away and get a white blood count that same day. If the white count has been lowered and you continue taking the drug, the infection could become fatal. However, a lowered white count will return to normal once you have stopped taking the drug.

Despite the fact that patients treated with anti-thyroid drugs have a decent chance of permanent remission, radioactive iodine (RAI) can be offered as treatment. In RAI, a radioactive iodine pill is given. The iodine concentrates in the thyroid, making it partially or fully inactive and reversing the hyperthyroidism. RAI is typically followed by an elevation in thyroid antibodies, which can further aggravate the autoimmune-related symptoms. According to experts, the majority of patients do become hypothyroid for life after RAI and while this is sometimes due to radiation-induced follicular damage, there are suggestions that this promotion of antibodies worsens the underlying thyroiditis and causes hypothyroidism.

Some innovative practitioners recommend a technique known as block replace therapy (BRT), which involves simultaneous use of anti-thyroid drugs to disable the overproduction and thyroid hormone replacement to suppress function and provide sufficient thyroid hormone.

Some doctors in the UK recommend surgery as the next step after anti-thyroid drugs. Increasingly, however, doctors are adopting the US model, and are viewing thyroidectomy only as a last resort after anti-thyroid drugs and RAI, or when the patient cannot tolerate anti-thyroid drugs or is not a good candidate for RAI (such as in a case of life-threatening hyperthyroidism during pregnancy). This surgery involves removal of all or part of the thyroid gland and can typically provide a permanent cure for hyperthyroidism. While the goal of surgery is to remove just enough of the gland so that thyroid production is normal, it's not often achieved. Determining how much of the gland to take is part science and part art. If too much is taken, then the patient can become hypothyroid. If all or part of the thyroid is surgically removed, hypothyroidism is still a strong possibility. There are several somewhat rare complications resulting from the surgery. One is vocal cord paralysis. Another is accidental removal of the parathyroid glands, which are located in the neck in back of the thyroid gland. Because the parathyroid glands regulate the amount of calcium in the body, their removal would result in low calcium levels.

GOITRE

A goitre is an enlargement of the thyroid. The condition can be detected by ultrasound or x-ray and may thicken the neck area visibly.

The thyroid usually becomes enlarged due to hyperthyroidism, hypothyroidism, autoimmune thyroid disease, multiple goitres or postpartum thyroiditis, an inflammation of the thyroid. It can also become enlarged due to deficiency or overconsumption of iodine.

Symptoms

You may have goitre if:

- your thyroid is enlarged, so your neck looks or feels swollen
- your neck or thyroid area is tender to the touch
- you have a tight feeling in your throat
- you frequently cough
- your voice is hoarse
- you have difficulty swallowing
- you have difficulty breathing and shortness of breath, especially at night
- you have a feeling that food is getting stuck in your throat.

If not caused by an autoimmune condition that triggers an inflamed thyroid, a goitre can be due to the level of iodine in your body. If there's too much iodine (e.g. from heart medications such as amiodarone), excess thyroid hormone can be produced and a hyperthyroid goitre can appear. If there is insufficient iodine in your diet, a hypothyroid goitre can develop. The use of iodized salt has wiped out the majority of goitres from iodine deficiency, but 10 to 20 per cent of goitres are still due to iodine deficiency.

Diagnosis

To self-test your thyroid, hold a mirror so that you can see the area of your neck just below the Adam's apple and right above the collarbone. This is the general location of your thyroid gland. Tip your head back while keeping this view of your neck and thyroid area in the mirror. Take a drink of water and swallow. As you swallow, look at your neck. Watch carefully for any bulges, enlargement, protrusions, or unusual appearances in this area. Repeat this process several times. If you see anything that appears unusual, contact your doctor right away. You may have an enlarged thyroid or a thyroid nodule and your thyroid should be evaluated. Be sure you don't get your Adam's apple confused with your thyroid gland. The Adam's apple is at the front of your neck; the thyroid is farther down and closer to your collarbone. Remember that this test is by no means conclusive and cannot rule out thyroid abnormalities. It's just helpful to identify a particularly enlarged thyroid or masses in the thyroid that warrant evaluation.

These steps can be involved in diagnosing goitre:

- examining and observing neck enlargement
- a blood test to determine if your thyroid is producing irregular amounts of thyroid hormone
- an antibody test to confirm an autoimmune disease, which may be the cause of your goitre
- an ultrasound test to evaluate the size of the enlargement
- a radioactive isotope thyroid scan to produce an image of the thyroid and provide visual information about the nature of the thyroid enlargement.

Treating Goitre

Treatment for goitre depends on how enlarged the thyroid has become, as well as other symptoms. Treatments can include:

- observation and monitoring, which is typically done if your goitre is not large and is not causing symptoms or thyroid dysfunction
- medications, including thyroid hormone replacement, which can help shrink your goitre, or aspirin or corticosteroid drugs to shrink thyroid inflammation
- surgery if the goitre is very large, continues to grow while on thyroid hormone or symptoms continue, or if the goitre is in a dangerous location (e.g. the windpipe or oesophagus) or is cosmetically unsightly. If the goitre contains suspicious nodules, this may also be reason for surgery.

THYROID NODULES

Sometimes your thyroid gland has lumps also known as *nodules*. These nodules, which can be solid or liquid filled, can be overactive and produce far too much thyroid hormone. They are called toxic nodules. When there are a lot of them, the condition is referred to as *a toxic multi-nodular goitre*.

Some of these nodules can result in hyperthyroidism. Thyroid nodules are actually fairly common. An estimated 1 in 12 to 15 women and 1 in 50 men has a thyroid nodule. More than 90 per cent of nodules are benign (except in pregnant women, in whom approximately 27 per cent of nodules are typically cancerous). It's vital to have your doctor examine a nodule as soon as you notice it.

Symptoms

Symptoms of thyroid nodules include palpitations, insomnia, weight loss, anxiety and tremors, which are all common in hyperthyroidism as well. Nodules can also trigger hypothyroidism and symptoms might include weight gain, fatigue and depression. Some people will cycle back and forth between hyperthyroid and hypothyroid symptoms. Others may have difficulty swallowing, feelings of fullness, pain or pressure in the neck, a hoarse voice and neck tenderness. Many people have nodules with no obvious symptoms related to thyroid dysfunction at all.

Diagnosis

Nodules are usually evaluated by:

- a blood test to determine whether they are producing thyroid hormone
- a radioactive thyroid scan, which looks at the reaction of the nodule to small amounts of radioactive material.
- an ultrasound of the thyroid to determine whether the nodule is solid or fluid filled
- a fine-needle aspiration or needle biopsy of the nodules to determine whether they may be cancerous.

Treating Thyroid Nodules

Depending on the results of the evaluation, nodules may be left alone and monitored periodically, assuming they aren't causing serious difficulty, treated with thyroid hormone replacement to help shrink them, or surgically removed if they are causing problems with breathing or if test results indicate a malignancy.

THYROID CANCER

Thyroid cancer is fairly uncommon and is considered very survivable, but according to the American Cancer Society, its numbers are on the rise. There are around 1,400 new cases of thyroid cancer diagnosed each year in the UK, and an estimated 3 men are diagnosed for each woman. It is estimated that more than 300 people die of thyroid cancer in the UK each year.

The treatment and prognosis for thyroid cancer depends on the type. Papillary and follicular thyroid cancer are the most common types; an estimated 80 to 90 per cent of all thyroid cancers fall into this category. Most of these cancers can be treated successfully when discovered early. Medullary thyroid carcinoma (MTC) makes up 5 to 10 per cent of all thyroid cancers. If discovered before it metastasizes to other parts of the body, it has a good cure rate. There are two types of medullary thyroid cancer: sporadic and familial. Anyone with a family history of MTC should take a blood test to measure calcitonin levels, which may indicate a strong possibility of a genetic predisposition. If found, a thyroidectomy may be performed as a preventive measure. Anaplastic thyroid carcinoma is quite rare, accounting for only 1 to 2 per cent of all thyroid cancers. It tends to be quite aggressive and is the least likely to respond to typical methods of treatment.

Symptoms

Although many patients are asymptomatic at first, possible symptoms of thyroid cancer include:

- a lump in your neck
- changes in your voice
- difficulty in breathing or swallowing
- lymph node swelling.

Diagnosis

The main diagnostic procedure for suspected thyroid cancer is a fine-needle aspiration (FNA) biopsy of the thyroid nodule. Using a needle, fluid and cells are removed from various parts of all nodules that can be felt and these samples are evaluated. Sometimes FNA tests are done with an ultrasound machine to help guide the needle into nodules that are too small to be felt. Between 60 and 80 per cent of FNA tests show that the nodule is benign. Only about 1 in 20 FNA tests reveals cancer. If a case is classified as suspicious, a surgical biopsy may be needed.

In everyone except pregnant women, a radioactive thyroid scan is frequently done in order to identify if the nodules are 'cold', meaning they have a greater potential to be cancerous.

Treating Thyroid Cancer

Under normal circumstances, patients with thyroid cancer have numerous treatments at their disposal such as radiation, chemotherapy and radioactive iodine treatment. Most, however, have surgery to remove part or all of the thyroid gland, rendering them hypothyroid for the rest of their lives. They must then take thyroid-replacement hormone, but their medication must keep their TSH levels low – nearly undetectable, actually – to help prevent a relapse of cancer.

There are treatments for all patients with cancer of the thyroid. The following types are commonly used:

- surgery (removal of the thyroid and the cancer)
- radiation therapy (to kill remaining cancer cells)
- hormone therapy (use of hormones to stop cancer cells from growing).

Surgery is the most common treatment of cancer for the thyroid. A doctor may remove the cancer using one of the following operations:

- Lobectomy removes only the side of the thyroid where the cancer is found. Lymph nodes in the area may be taken out (biopsied) to see if they contain cancer.
- Near-total thyroidectomy removes all of the thyroid except for a small part.
- Total thyroidectomy removes the entire thyroid.
- Lymph node dissection removes lymph nodes in the neck that contain cancer.

Radiation for cancer of the thyroid may come from a machine outside the body (external radiation therapy), or more commonly from drinking a liquid that contains radioactive iodine (RAI). Because the thyroid takes up iodine, the radioactive iodine collects in any thyroid tissue remaining in the body and kills the cancer cells.

Hormone therapy uses thyroid hormone replacement drugs to stop cancer cells from growing. In treating cancer of the thyroid, the thyroid hormone replacement can be used to deactivate any remaining thyroid tissue in the body.

Overall, the prognosis for thyroid cancer is quite good. However, survivors need to be vigilant in case of a reoccurrence. Regular check-ups and scans by their doctors are in order.

THYROID DISEASE RISKS AND SYMPTOMS CHECKLIST

THYROID DISEASE RISK FACTORS

Age/Gender

- ❏ Age over 60
- ❏ Female

Medical History

- ❏ Past history of thyroid problems
- ❏ Had radioactive iodine (RAI) treatment in the past
- ❏ Had surgery for goitre, nodules, Hashimoto's disease, or thyroid cancer
- ❏ Family history of thyroid problems
- ❏ Past history of autoimmune disease
- ❏ Family history of autoimmune disease
- ❏ Currently a smoker
- ❏ Formerly a smoker
- ❏ Allergies or sensitivity to gluten

Related Conditions

Currently or in the past diagnosed with the following diseases or conditions:

- ❏ Other pituitary or endocrine disease (e.g. diabetes, pituitary tumour, polycystic ovary syndrome [PCOS], endometriosis, premature menopause)
- ❏ Chronic fatigue syndrome/ME
- ❏ Fibromyalgia
- ❏ Carpal tunnel syndrome/tendonitis/plantar fasciitis
- ❏ Mitral valve prolapse syndrome (MVPS) (heart murmur, palpitations)
- ❏ Epstein-Barr Virus (EBV)
- ❏ Glandular fever/Mononucleosis
- ❏ Depression
- ❏ Infertility, recurrent miscarriage
- ❏ Coeliac disease/gluten intolerance

Radiation Exposure History

- ❏ Work at a nuclear plant
- ❏ Live near or downwind from a nuclear plant
- ❏ Lived near or downwind from the Chernobyl nuclear disaster in 1986
- ❏ Had radiation treatments to neck area (e.g. for Hodgkin's disease, nasal radium therapy, radiation to tonsils and neck area)

Medications/Supplements

- ❏ Currently or formerly treated with lithium
- ❏ Currently or formerly treated with amiodarone
- ❏ Currently taking supplemental iodine, kelp, bladder wrack and/or bugleweed

Dietary Factors

- ❏ Live in an iodine-deficient area, such as the US Goitre Belt, Ireland, or other iodine-deficient regions including: Belgium, Denmark, France, Germany, Greece, Hungary, Italy, Romania, Slovenia, Spain, Turkey
- ❏ Have significantly cut back or eliminated iodized salt from the diet
- ❏ Heavy consumer of soy products
- ❏ Heavy consumer of raw goitrogenic foods – Brussels sprouts, rutabaga, turnips, kohlrabi, radishes, cauliflower, African cassava, millet, babassu (a palm-tree coconut fruit popular in Brazil and Africa), cabbage and kale

Toxic Exposures

- ❏ Work at a rocket fuel, fireworks or explosives production plant
- ❏ Live in an area where there is currently or formerly a rocket fuel, fireworks or explosives production plant
- ❏ Excessively exposed to mercury
- ❏ High exposure to pesticides
- ❏ Use fluoridated water
- ❏ Regularly have dental fluoride treatments

Hormonal Status

- ❏ Currently in the perimenopause
- ❏ Currently in the menopause
- ❏ Postmenopausal
- ❏ Had a baby within the past year

Trauma/Injury

- ❏ Have had serious trauma to the neck, such as whiplash from a car accident or a broken neck

THYROID DISEASE SYMPTOMS
Energy/Mood/Thinking

- ❏ Exhaustion, fatigue
- ❏ Depressed, moody, sad
- ❏ Difficulty concentrating
- ❏ Thinking is fuzzy; have difficulty concentrating, difficulty remembering

Anxiety/Panic

❑ Heart palpitations
❑ Tremors in hands
❑ Panic attacks
❑ Erratic behaviour
❑ Anxiety, irritability, nervousness or panic attacks

Temperature

❑ Sensitive to cold and cold hands and/or feet
❑ Sweating more than usual, feeling hot when others are not

Weight

❑ Inappropriate weight gain, or having difficulty losing weight despite changes in diet and exercise
❑ Rapid weight loss, inability to gain weight

Hair/Nails/Skin

❑ Dry, tangled and/or coarse hair
❑ Fine and brittle hair
❑ Hair loss, maybe even from the outer part of the eyebrows
❑ Dry and/or brittle nails
❑ Dry skin
❑ Thickening of skin in shin area of legs
❑ Itching, prickly hot skin, rashes and hives (urticaria)

Muscles/Joints/Nerves

❑ Muscle and joint pains and aches
❑ Carpal tunnel syndrome, or tendonitis in arms and legs
❑ Soles of the feet are painful
❑ Muscle pain and weakness, especially in the upper arms and thighs

Sex/Reproduction/Fertility/Menstruation

❑ Abnormally low sex drive
❑ Unexplained infertility, or recurrent miscarriages with no obvious explanation
❑ Menstrual period is heavier than normal, or period is longer than it used to be, or comes more frequently
❑ Periods have stopped
❑ Periods very light and infrequent
❑ Difficulty getting pregnant

Digestion

❑ Constipation
❑ Diarrhoea

Neck/Throat

- ❑ Full or sensitive feeling in the neck
- ❑ Raspy, hoarse voice
- ❑ Enlarged thyroid
- ❑ Neck looks or feels swollen
- ❑ Neck or thyroid area may be tender to the touch
- ❑ Tight feeling in the throat
- ❑ Frequent coughing
- ❑ Difficulty swallowing
- ❑ Difficulty breathing and shortness of breath, especially at night
- ❑ Feeling that food is stuck in throat

Vital Signs

- ❑ Rapid pulse
- ❑ Elevated blood pressure
- ❑ Slow pulse
- ❑ Low blood pressure

Eyes

- ❑ Double vision, scratchy eyes, dry eyes
- ❑ Eyes are bulging or more whites are showing than usual

Other Symptoms

- ❑ Lymph node swelling
- ❑ Face, eyes, arms, or legs are abnormally swollen or puffy
- ❑ Cholesterol levels are high and not responsive to diet and medication
- ❑ Allergies worsening
- ❑ Frequent infections, including yeast infections, oral fungus, thrush or sinus infections
- ❑ Shortness of breath, sometimes difficulty drawing a full breath, or a need to yawn
- ❑ Difficulty falling asleep or staying asleep

CHAPTER 2

Thyroid Diagnosis, Treatment and Optimization Challenges

If you don't want to be the horses' hoofprints,
you got to be the hooves.

— BRUCE COCKBURN

For some of you, just recognizing the symptoms of a thyroid problem will trigger a visit to the doctor, conventional tests will reveal your thyroid problem, the doctor will give you a prescription, and you'll be on your way to feeling better and normalizing your metabolism and weight. Unfortunately, for some of you, getting a doctor who will test, diagnose and properly treat your thyroid condition may not be as smooth a process as you'd hope, for a number of reasons.

CHALLENGES TO DIAGNOSIS
Inability to Get Tested or Diagnosed

You may find that your doctor isn't willing to test your thyroid. Sometimes it's because the test was your idea, which can threaten a doctor's ego or sense of control. Or your doctor may be afraid that you want thyroid drugs as weight-loss aids. Some doctors in private practice, and even on the NHS, face restrictions or financial disincentives to order lab tests. Finally, some doctors are simply not particularly aware of or informed about thyroid disease. Some patients have even reported that their doctors refused to perform thyroid tests, saying totally off-base things such as:

- 'You're only in your 20s. Only older people get thyroid disease.'
- 'You just had a baby and if you had a thyroid problem, you wouldn't have been able to get pregnant.'
- 'I can tell by looking at you that you don't have a thyroid problem.'
- 'I don't feel anything in your neck, so your thyroid is fine.'
- 'You're a man and men almost never get thyroid problems.'

In other cases, you may describe your thyroid symptoms but end up with another diagnosis. Say 'fatigue, weight gain and moodiness' to many doctors and you'll leave the office not with a thyroid test but with a prescription for an antidepressant. Some researchers estimate that at least 15 per cent of those diagnosed with depression are actually suffering from undiagnosed hypothyroidism.

Or you may be told 'It's your hormones' (which in essence it is, but they're talking about the *wrong* hormones here!). Or you may be told you're experiencing the effects of getting older, working too hard, normal postpartum symptoms, or lack of exercise. If you describe feelings of anxiety and weight loss, you may, as some young women with hyperthyroidism have experienced, be labelled as anorexic or bulimic.

When faced with a doctor who is oblivious or resistant to what may be very obvious thyroid symptoms, or won't test when asked, the best option is to find another doctor, even if you have to pay for it yourself. But if you have no options, here are a few tips:

- Be persistent but unemotional. Ask for a thyroid test. Show the doctor articles about thyroid disease that reflect your symptoms.
- Quantify your symptoms as much as possible. Many people go into the doctor saying, 'I'm just so tired and I can't stand it. I'm gaining weight!' The doctor's response is likely to be, 'Get more sleep, get off the couch, exercise and don't eat so much.' Rather than saying, 'I'm tired,' explain that you need to sleep 10 hours a night instead of 8 hours and you're still exhausted by dinnertime. Instead of saying, 'I can't lose weight,' say, 'I'm eating 1,500 calories per day on a low-fat diet, doing 4 hours a week on the treadmill and 2 hours a week of muscle-building exercise and I'm gaining 2 pounds a week.'
- Bring your Risks and Symptoms Checklist to your doctor (see Chapter 1) and ask that it be included in your medical records after the doctor

signs and dates it, indicating that he/she has read and discussed it. Keep a signed copy for yourself. If relevant, send a copy to the insurance company's consumer liaison, along with your request that testing be approved.

- Write a letter that states the various reasons you have requested thyroid testing and the fact that this doctor has refused. Insist that the doctor sign it, place a copy in your records and give you a copy. (You can then use this copy to argue for a referral to another doctor if needed.)

If you take these steps, you'll probably get the tests you need. It may seem ridiculous that you have to struggle to get standard medical tests and treatment, but it's your health that is at stake, so keep fighting.

Test Value Changes

Your doctor may not be up to date on the latest thyroid recommendations regarding revised lab standards for the thyroid-stimulating hormone (TSH) test, which is considered by most conventional doctors to be the primary diagnostic tool. Many doctors are still operating according to the old 'normal' range and therefore will inaccurately rule out thyroid conditions. Take a look at the guidelines at http://www.nacb.org/lmpg/thyroid_LMPG_PDF.stm and share them with your GP.

Borderline Levels

Your TSH level may be borderline. In that situation, despite your symptoms, your doctor may refuse to treat you. Don't accept a response of wait-and-see. Ask for the actual number and ask for the normal range for the lab where your blood was tested. Show your doctor your Risks and Symptoms Checklist and ask about a trial course of treatment to see if your symptoms improve. If your doctor is so number-obsessed that it's like talking to an accountant instead of a healthcare practitioner, start looking for a new doctor.

Over-reliance on the TSH Test

Some doctors believe that only the TSH test is necessary and refuse to order free T4 or free T3 tests. The problem is that some people who have a borderline TSH level may have changes to free T4 and free T3 that point to a diagnosable thyroid problem. Without those additional numbers, however, a normal or borderline TSH will not reveal the underlying problem. Push for additional testing, or consider finding a doctor who will order the tests for you.

Failure to Test for Antibodies

Even though autoimmune problems are most frequently the cause of thyroid conditions, some doctors do not routinely conduct the antibody tests that diagnose autoimmune thyroid disease. This presents a problem because elevated thyroid antibodies, even in the presence of normal TSH levels, mean that you have autoimmune thyroid disease and that your thyroid is in the process of autoimmune dysfunction. The dysfunction may not be significant enough to register as an abnormal TSH level, but the presence of antibodies may generate symptoms and is predictive of thyroid problems down the road.

The practice of treating patients who have Hashimoto's thyroiditis but normal-range TSH levels is supported by a study reported in the March 2001 issue of the journal *Thyroid*. In this study, German researchers found that treatment with Synthetic thyroxine for Hashimoto's autoimmune thyroiditis – where TSH had not yet elevated beyond normal range – could actually reduce the chance and severity of autoimmune disease progression. The researchers speculated that such treatment might even be able to stop the progression of Hashimoto's disease or prevent the development of hypothyroidism.

Some doctors will not, however, treat patients who present clinical symptoms of hypothyroidism and test positive for Hashimoto's antibodies but have a normal TSH level. You may have to interview endocrinologists, as well as holistic doctors, osteopaths and other practitioners, to find one who will treat you if you have a normal TSH level, with thyroid antibodies and symptoms.

Normal Levels but Low T3/T4/T3 Conversion Problems

One of the most difficult situations is having an underlying thyroid problem that does not show up on standard thyroid blood tests. You may have a family history of thyroid disease or a number of thyroid symptoms – even a low basal body temperature – but you have TSH, free T4, free T3 and antibody levels that are normal. What you may be experiencing is *thyroid hormone resistance*, where your body is capable of producing thyroid hormone, but nutritional and metabolic dysfunctions have made your tissues resistant to that hormone. This is similar to the better-known concept of insulin resistance, where your body produces enough insulin but your cells become resistant to it, so your body loses its ability to respond to it.

You may also have thyroid hormone conversion problems, where you have enough T4 and T3 in the bloodstream, but the organs and tissues are not effectively converting the inactive T4 into the active T3 that you need at the cellular level. In both cases you may show normal circulating levels, but you are hypothyroid at the level of your tissues, organs and cells.

Thyroid hormone resistance and conversion problems are very difficult to diagnose with blood tests. Some practitioners perform a reverse T3 test that measures the conversion of T4 to reverse T3 – an inactive form of T3. This typically occurs when the body is under stress and is cause for treatment, according to some practitioners. This test is considered irrelevant by some practitioners, however.

The bottom line is that if you suspect thyroid resistance or conversion problems, you will need a practitioner who is skilled in clinical, observational diagnosis and who, in the face of normal blood test values, will still be willing to try you on a course of thyroid treatment if you have observable signs of hypothyroidism. Typically, this would be a holistic or alternative medicine practitioner with expertise working with thyroid disease and other difficult-to-diagnose conditions.

OPTIMIZING YOUR THYROID TREATMENT

If I seem to be focusing on hypothyroidism, it's because it's ultimately the end result for most thyroid patients. For example, with Hashimoto's thyroiditis patients, the thyroid typically burns itself out over time, becoming less able to produce thyroid hormone, thus leaving most patients hypothyroid. With Graves' disease and hyperthyroidism, most doctors rush to administer radioactive iodine (RAI), which leaves patients without a functional thyroid. They end up hypothyroid even if they started out with an overactive gland. Many doctors do not explain this fully to patients when they recommend RAI treatment.

With thyroid nodules and goitre, surgery may be performed to remove all or part of the thyroid. The end result is often hypothyroidism. And for thyroid cancer, almost all patients have their thyroid removed entirely, leaving them completely hypothyroid and reliant on outside thyroid hormone replacement.

However you have got there, if you are battling weight issues, once you become hypothyroid it's a shared battle. After getting diagnosed and treated, the first step is to optimize your thyroid hormone replacement treatment.

If you are still suffering from thyroid symptoms and finding it difficult or impossible to lose weight, or you're gaining weight even though you're on a healthy diet and exercise programme, there's a good chance that your thyroid treatment is not optimized. A number of situations can contribute to less than optimal thyroid treatment:

- problems with production of T4
- problems with conversion of T4 to T3
- problems with the cells' ability to take up T3.

Any of these problems can interfere with optimal thyroid function and disrupt metabolism. Here are some questions you can consider that address the various concerns relating to optimal thyroid function.

Are You on the Right Brand of Medication for You?

Some people simply do not feel well on particular brands, and changing brands seems to help. With several brands available, you may wish to discuss a change with your doctor.

Do You Need the Addition of T3?

Some people do not feel their best and find it difficult to lose weight without the addition of a second thyroid hormone known as T3. T3 is the active thyroid hormone. Usually the body converts T4 to T3, but nutritional deficiencies, toxins and a variety of other physiological factors may prevent the body from accomplishing that conversion process properly, leaving you deficient in this most important thyroid hormone. In one research study, experts found that among a group of 100 obese patients, more than 90 per cent of those studied had T3 levels that were below the mean. So it's clear that low T3 or inability to convert T4 to T3 may contribute to weight gain or difficulty losing weight.

While it's a controversial topic that is under increasing study by various experts, some doctors believe that supplemental T3 may be a solution to help optimize thyroid treatment for some patients. They add T3 in one of several ways:

- via a prescription brand of T3 drug
- via a compounded time-released T3
- via a combination synthetic drug which includes both T4 and T3
- via natural desiccated thyroid, which also includes a full array of natural thyroid hormones including T3

Key point? Check with your GP about whether supplemental T3 might be helpful for you.

Would Natural Thyroid Help?

Some practitioners believe that certain patients simply do best on natural desiccated thyroid derived from the thyroid gland of pigs. These products are prescription thyroid drugs that have been in use for a century. Alternative experts believe that these drugs, which provide T4, T3, T2, T1 and other thyroid hormones and nutritional elements, more closely resemble human thyroid hormone than the synthetics and report that their patients feel better on them. Keep in mind that many conventional doctors feel that these drugs are out of date and won't prescribe them, so you may need to find a holistic or alternative practitioner.

Kim describes her experiences with natural thyroid:

> I convinced my doctor to put me on the natural thyroid medication rather than the synthetic that I had been on for years. The very first day with the natural, I felt so much better; I felt I could actually open my eyes. I also had more energy and after not being able to lose weight and knowing I was eating properly, the first month I lost 16 pounds, doing the same things and eating the same things that I had done before. When my doctor saw the results from my blood test and my weight loss and my blood pressure, he was very impressed and very proud of me. He said he would definitely keep me on the natural and that I am just one of the people that it works better for.

Are You at the Optimal Dosage/TSH for You?

While the normal range for TSH lab tests is established for each lab, where you personally feel best will vary. A study reported in the *Journal of Clinical Endocrinology and Metabolism* found that the mean TSH level for people who don't have a thyroid condition is 1.5. And the American Association of Clinical Endocrinologists has stated that TSH levels above 3 would be considered potential evidence of a developing thyroid problem. So it's no wonder that if your TSH is on the higher end of normal for you, you may find it hard to lose weight. Check your most recent blood test results and consult with your GP about whether a slight increase in medication dosage and a reduction in TSH would be better for your health.

Allie, who is 50, started having a weight problem around the time she hit 40. She also had a laundry list of symptoms, including dry skin, hot flushes, memory loss and low sex drive. Her doctor decided it was the menopause and depression. Allie kept insisting on a thyroid test. She was finally tested and diagnosed as hypothyroid at age 48. Her symptoms continued and she insisted on more blood work. Her TSH level was 5.2, which according to Allie's doctor was normal.

> I insisted that, knowing my body, it was too high for me. He was quite adamant that my problem was not my thyroid, but that I needed to admit that it was depression and that I had all the symptoms. When I told him that all of my symptoms were from a low thyroid problem and that the latest count just wasn't compatible with my body and that I wasn't depressed, his answer was, 'I'll bet 95 per cent of the people in the psychiatric ward say the same thing.'

Allie finally saw another doctor, who said she was being undertreated and upped her dosage of thyroid hormone replacement. She's feeling dramatically better.

One other little-known issue for thyroid patients is the seasonal variation in thyroid function. A number of studies show that TSH naturally rises during colder months and drops to a low normal or even a hyperthyroid level in the warmest months. Some doctors adjust for this by prescribing slightly increased dosages during colder months and reducing dosages during warm periods. Most, however, are not aware of this seasonal fluctuation, leaving patients suffering with worsening hypothyroidism symptoms during colder months, or going through warmer months suffering with hyperthyroidism symptoms due to slight overdosage. This seasonal fluctuation becomes more pronounced in older people, particularly in cold climates. Twice-yearly tests at a minimum during winter and summer months can help assess fluctuations and guide seasonal dosage modifications if needed.

Are You Taking Your Medication Properly?

There are a number of guidelines on how to take thyroid hormone properly to ensure that you are absorbing the drug and receiving the maximum possible benefit:

- Don't take your thyroid hormone replacement drug within 4 hours of taking calcium supplements or calcium-fortified juice. This includes antacids in liquid or tablet form, which also contain calcium and can delay or reduce the absorption of your thyroid hormone.
- Don't take thyroid hormone replacement drugs within 4 hours of taking any supplements that contain iron, including ante-natal vitamins, which are usually high in iron.
- Try to take your thyroid hormone around the same time each day. For best results, maximum absorption and minimum interference from food, fibre and supplements, doctors recommend taking it in the morning on an empty stomach, about an hour before eating.
- If you need to take your thyroid hormone with food, be consistent and *always* take it with food.
- If you start or stop a high-fibre diet while you are on thyroid hormone, have your thyroid function retested around 6 to 8 weeks after your dietary change. High-fibre diets can change the speed of thyroid drug absorption and you may require a dosage adjustment. You should also be consistent about your daily fibre intake. Don't have 10 grams one day, 30 grams the next day and so on, or you're risking erratic absorption.

NUTRITION AND SUPPLEMENTS FOR THYROID FUNCTION
Multivitamins

A high-potency multivitamin is essential for thyroid patients. Look for one that has high amounts of vitamins B, C and E and a good range of minerals. One that I particularly like is Dr Jacob Teitelbaum's formulation known as Daily Energy Enfusion (see Appendix A). Dr Teitelbaum's formula does contain some iodine, however, so you may want to slightly reduce your daily dosage if you are iodine sensitive. The vitamin comes as a flavourful powdered drink along with one B vitamin capsule; this replaces more than 30 vitamins and supplement pills each day. Dr Teitelbaum's formula does not include iron or calcium, so it can be taken at the same time as thyroid pills.

Another good option if you want an iodine- and iron-free antioxidant multivitamin is Advanced Nutritional System's Rainbow Light: Complete Antioxidant Multivitamin and Advanced Nutritional System's Rainbow

Light Iron-Free Complete Nutritional System Multivitamin. The first is a high-power multivitamin and the second adds green foods, herbs and enzymes.

Probiotics

Probiotics are supplements that contain live bacteria – the 'good' bacteria found in fermented foods such as miso and dairy products such as yogurt and some cheeses – that we are meant to have in sufficient quantities in our intestinal system. One of the more well-known probiotic bacterium is *acidophilus*, the live cultures found in yogurt. According to a report in the *European Journal of Clinical Nutrition*, the probiotic bacteria known as *Bifidobacterium lactis* HN019 boosts the activity of various disease-killing immune system cells in healthy adults. Probiotics help proper digestive functioning, which enhances the immune system. They also kill off harmful bacteria, having an antibiotic effect by fighting off various types of infection. You can take yogurt, but the concentration of live cultures in yogurt is not high enough to get a substantial effect, so a probiotic supplement is your best option. Some probiotic supplements can be expensive and require refrigeration, but I recommend a patented formula from Enzymatic Therapies, the Probiotic Pearl. This tiny pearl-shaped supplement contains a guaranteed level of live bacteria in the millions, is very inexpensive and requires no refrigeration.

Zinc

Zinc is important for thyroid hormone production and conversion, and 15 to 25 mg of zinc a day can help ensure optimum zinc delivery to the thyroid. Zinc, along with selenium, can also help prevent the decline of T3 when you are on a lower-calorie diet.

Selenium

Research has shown that selenium is an important mineral for thyroid function. It activates an enzyme responsible for controlling thyroid function by the conversion of T4 to T3. Stress and injury appear to make the body particularly thyroid responsive and selenium deficient. Supplemental selenium appears to offset the effect of high iodine intake on thyroid function. A 1997 study suggested that high intake of iodine when selenium is deficient may permit thyroid damage. Selenium supplementation has been shown to reduce inflammation in patients with autoimmune thyroiditis. Too much selenium can be dangerous, so multivitamin and additional supplementation should not exceed 400 mcg per day.

L-tyrosine

L-tyrosine is a known precursor to thyroid hormone and low levels can make it difficult for the thyroid to function properly. It is a common component of many thyroid support supplements that combine several supplements into one capsule. Tyrosine supplements at the level of 85 to 170 mg a day may be helpful to the thyroid.

Guggul

Z-guggulsterone – known as guggul – is derived from the plant commiphora mukul and has been used in Ayurvedic medicine as an anti-inflammatory, anti-obesity, thyroid-stimulating and cholesterol-lowering agent. Guggul is considered particularly important for prevention of a sluggish metabolism and studies have shown that Z-guggulsterone has the ability to increase the thyroid's ability to take up the enzymes it needs for effective hormone conversion. It also increases the oxygen uptake in muscles. Some people find that guggul is overstimulating, so you need to be careful with this supplement.

Essential Fatty Acids

Essential fatty acids (EFAs) cannot be produced in the body, so you must get them through diet or supplements. The key essential fatty acids include:

- Omega-3/alpha-linolenic acid (ALA), eicosapentaenoic acid (EPA), docosahexaenoic acid (DHA) - found in fresh fish from cold, deep oceans (e.g. mackerel, tuna, herring, flounder, sardines, salmon, rainbow trout, bass), linseed oil, flaxseeds and oil, blackcurrant and pumpkin seeds, cod liver oil, shrimp, oysters, leafy greens, soybeans, walnuts, wheat germ, fresh sea vegetables such as seaweed, and fish oil. Usually, your body can convert ALA into EPA, then into DHA.

- Omega-6/linoleic acid/gamma-linolenic acid (GLA) – found in breast milk, sesame, safflower, cotton and sunflower seeds and oil, corn and corn oil, soybeans, raw nuts, legumes, leafy greens, blackcurrant seeds, evening primrose oil, borage oil, spirulina, soybeans, lecithin. Linoleic acid in omega-6 can be converted into GLA.

According to Dr Udo Erasmus, author of *Fats That Heal, Fats That Kill*, imbalances and deficiencies in essential fatty acids are the cause, a trigger, or a contributing factor to many diseases and conditions. Addressing those deficiencies through proper foods or the use of healthy oils can have huge implications for health. He believes that essential fatty acids are critical to thyroid function because (1) they are required for the integrity of the structure for every membrane of every cell, (2) they increase energy levels in the cell, and (3) there is some evidence that essential fatty acids, especially omega-3s, improve the body's ability to detect and respond to thyroid hormone effectively.

Erasmus also points to the role that EFAs play in preventing and reducing inflammation. In particular, essential fatty acids make hormone-like eicosanoids that regulate immune and inflammatory responses and omega-3s in particular have anti-inflammatory effects that can slow autoimmune damage. Inflammation of the thyroid – known as goitre – is central to many cases of autoimmune thyroid disease and inflammation is generally seen in almost all autoimmune diseases.

Erasmus believes that if proteins are the juice, fats are the insulators, not just of nerves but of cells and membranes. Protein reactions lead to inflammation, allergies and autoimmune disease. Essential fatty acids seem to help prevent the proteins from becoming hyperactive and triggering these various immune reactions.

Nutritional expert Ann Louise Gittleman, author of *Eat Fat, Lose Weight* and the best-selling book *The Fat Flush Plan*, believes that good fats are essential to good health and weight loss and that today's low-fat diets are counterproductive. Gittleman says, 'Even as we have cut back on fat in the last decade, weight has steadily increased, an average of 8 pounds per person. We may be eating less fat, but we are eating more calories.' Ultimately, Gittleman, like many other nutritional experts, believes that if you include good fats in the diet, you rev up the body's fat-burning potential and you stay full longer, so you eat fewer calories without feeling hungry.

Overall, EFA supplements appear to be an important part of any weight-loss effort for the following reasons:

- EFAs help your body metabolize stored fat more efficiently.
- EFAs help reduce the output of inflammatory markers from fat tissue and reduce inflammation in joints and muscles.
- EFAs can help reduce insulin resistance.
- EFAs can help balance blood sugar.
- EFAs can help reduce appetite.
- EFAs can improve cholesterol levels.
- EFAs can help reduce blood pressure.
- EFAs help keep hair, skin and nails healthy.

In addition to adding more of the foods that contain these essential fatty acids, some of the ways you can add EFAs to your diet include:

- Omega-3/fish oil supplements – go for a decent-tasting oil or a 'burpless' capsule (Enzymatic Therapies' Eskimo Oil is my favourite)
- Omega-3/flaxseeds and flaxseed oil – you can add flaxseed oils to meals, either in the oil form or as capsules. Some people like to make salad dressings out of the oil or add it to soups. Taking flaxseed oil with each meal helps slow down digestion and modulate blood sugar fluctuations (which helps with insulin levels).
- Omega-6/evening primrose oil, borage oil – these are usually taken as supplements.

GLA is thought to help activate brown fat and boost metabolic efficiency. Gittleman is an advocate of evening primrose oil.

> In my private practice, I have seen women and men benefit time and time again from the addition of omega fats to their weight-loss plans. Many of my clients who have had at least 10 pounds or more of weight to lose have reported staggeringly dramatic results with four to eight capsules of 500 mg evening primrose oil [daily].

If you want to include a healthy balance of EFAs, think about a product that includes a balance of oils, such as the Atkins formulated Essential Oils Supplement, or Udo Erasmus' Udo's Oil products.

OTHER THYROID SUPPORT ALTERNATIVES
Watch Goitrogens

Goitrogens are products and foods that promote goitre formation and can act like anti-thyroid drugs in disabling the thyroid and causing hypothyroidism. Specifically, goitrogens inhibit the body's ability to use iodine, block the process by which iodine becomes the thyroid hormones T4 and T3, inhibit the actual secretion of thyroid hormone and disrupt the peripheral conversion of T4 to T3.

If you are hypothyroid due to thyroidectomy, you don't have to be particularly concerned about goitrogens. If you still have a thyroid, however, you need to be careful not to eat goitrogens in large quantities. The enzymes involved in the formation of goitrogenic materials in plants can be partially destroyed by cooking. Eating moderate amounts of goitrogenic foods, raw or cooked, is probably not a problem for most people. The following list contains some of the more common and potent goitrogens (particularly when consumed raw):

African cassava	Babassu (palm-tree coconut fruit found
Broccoli	in Brazil and Africa)
Cabbage	Brussels sprouts
Kale	Cauliflower
Millet	Kohlrabi
Radishes	Mustard
Soy products	Rutabaga
Watercress	Turnips

Salt - no
Sea Salt yes

Reduce Toxic Exposures

Fluoride has been used in the treatment of hyperthyroidism, meaning that it has the ability to suppress thyroid function. In one study, it was shown that 2.3 to 4.5 mg of fluoride per day was a successful treatment for hyperthyroidism. In areas where water is fluoridated, typical fluoride intake ranges from 1.6 to 6.6 mg/day, which in some cases exceeds the dosage used for medical treatment of hyperthyroidism. What can you do? Drink bottled water that is not fluoridated. Use a fluoride-free toothpaste. And do not get fluoride treatments at the dentist. These treatments have not been clearly demonstrated to be helpful in adults for reducing or preventing cavities.

The rocket fuel/explosives manufacturing by-product, perchlorate, a chemical that is known to disrupt thyroid function and cause other health problems, is increasingly the focus of public, media and government attention. Perchlorate has contaminated areas of the US water supply, most commonly in the western part of the country. Eating lettuce or other vegetables and fruits irrigated with perchlorate-contaminated water may expose some consumers to high levels of the toxin. Perchlorate is also a component of fertilizers and can contaminate foods grown with them. There's not much you can do to avoid eating perchlorate-contaminated foods, except to grow your own produce and water it with water that you've had tested for perchlorate contamination. If you drink well water, you should also have that water tested and if you live in an area near a current or former production facility for rockets, explosives or fireworks, consider having your water independently tested. Most importantly, become aware of the issues and monitor the status of perchlorate legislation by monitoring the comprehensive site: www.perchlorate.org.

Mercury exposure comes through dental fillings and some fish. Mercury levels can be tested by a holistic practitioner or nutritionist using hair analysis. If you have excessive levels of mercury, some experts recommend *chelation* – the process of helping the body excrete excess metals and minerals. This can be done through intravenous infusion or herbal supplements. In some cases, practitioners recommend removing mercury fillings and replacing them with composite materials that contain no mercury. This is controversial, not least because it can be very expensive. Some patients, however, have reported that their thyroid problems and other symptoms were greatly relieved with removal of mercury fillings.

Treat Infections

Infection is also thought to be a trigger for some thyroid problems. The food-borne bacteria *Yersinia enterocolitica*, for example, has been associated with the production and elevated levels of thyroid antibodies, which is a sign of autoimmune thyroid disease.

A lab analysis by Great Smokies (see Appendix A) can help detect intestinal bacterial overgrowth which could be contributing to underlying immune system problems that may be fuelling your thyroid condition. Bacteria are typically treated with antibiotics, or a special diet, nutritional supplements and herbs that function in an antibiotic-like capacity.

Yoga

In addition to the overall health benefits of yoga, this ancient art and science of mind–body wellness offers several specific practices focused on the thyroid. A particular yoga breathing exercise is designed to help the thyroid and the throat chakra. Breathe in through your nose, focusing the inhalation towards the back of your throat. Your throat should feel slightly closed or blocked while you perform this breathing exercise. Mentally, you should try to feel as if you are taking in the air through the front of your throat. Do this several times a day but not for long periods, as it might make you dizzy.

A specific *asana* – or pose – is also thought to be of great benefit to the thyroid. The half-shoulder stand (*viparit karani mudra*) and shoulder stand (*sarvangasan*) positions both invert and stimulate the thyroid. The shoulder stand is considered one of the most powerful positions in yoga. In addition to helping the thyroid, it is thought to prolong life through its effect on the metabolism and pranic energy.

In a shoulder stand, you lie flat on your back, keep your legs together and raise them up until they are at a right angle to your shoulders/neck, perpendicular to the floor, chin tucked into your chest, resting the weight of your body on your shoulders and elbows, arms supporting your hips. In a half-shoulder stand, the legs don't need to be as straight as in a full shoulder stand. Work up to a daily session of a full 2 minutes by starting with two or three shorter sessions. As an alternative, you can support your legs on a wall or chair, if the shoulder stand position is too difficult.

Guided Chakra Visualization/Affirmation

In the area of energy work, there is a guided visualization and meditation that can be done to help tune and balance the thyroid. Sit in a comfortable upright position (in a chair or on a sofa, or in a cross-legged yoga lotus position), eyes closed. Take a few deep, cleansing breaths. The harmonic colour for the thyroid is blue, so you should visualize a bright blue beam of light coming down through the top of your head and going right to your thyroid. Feel the blue energy infusing every cell of your thyroid, throat and neck. Visualize the blue beam of energy enhancing the thyroid and curing its underactivity. Feel the blue light softly spreading all around your neck and throat. Now, say out loud, 'My thyroid is energized and is working perfectly. I am safe and loved and filled with the energy of the Universe.'

CONTROVERSIES
The Iodine Controversy

Iodization of salt and foods has helped eliminate epidemic goitre and cretinism in areas that are iodine deficient, but excess inorganic iodine may also contribute to thyroid imbalances. One gram of salt contains 76 mcg of iodine, and we need approximately 100 mcg daily. The average person actually consumes as much as 3 grams of salt, however, so you may well be overdosing on iodine.

Some alternative practitioners automatically recommend iodine or iodine-containing herbs or supplements such as bladder wrack and bugleweed supplementation when they hear 'thyroid problem'. But do you need this supplemental iodine? In all likelihood, no. A study reported in the *Journal of Clinical Endocrinology and Metabolism* in late 1998 indicated that the percentage of Americans with a low intake of iodine had more than quadrupled since the 1970s. Yet statistically only one in nine of us is iodine deficient, so in all likelihood you are getting enough. It's even more likely that you're getting too much.

One way to cut back on iodine intake is to stop buying commercially iodized salt (salt that has potassium iodide) and use sea salt instead. An added plus is that sea salt tastes better!

However, if you are iodine deficient, this can factor into your thyroid problem. You can always have a doctor or nutritionist test for iodine deficiency, but a short course of iodine may be an adequate self-test to see whether you need this supplement. Or you can consider the input of Drs Richard and Karilee Shames, authors of *Thyroid Power*, who say,

> If you are a person who never consumes fast food, avoids salt like the plague, doesn't eat much seafood and feels that sea vegetables are for fish, and especially if you live more than 100 miles from any coast, then you might well consider supplementation with iodine.

Some alternative and conventional practitioners have found that iodine or iodine-containing herbal products aggravate hypothyroid symptoms. I have tried iodine on numerous occasions and, within a day or two, I always feel exhausted, with a swollen, irritated neck. After a week, I'm barely functional. I can tolerate the small amount of iodine in a multivitamin, and I eat sea vegetables and iodine-rich foods like seaweed/sushi or shellfish without any problem, however, so perhaps the obstacle is a sensitivity to processed iodine rather than the iodine found naturally in food.

Soy

There is a definite debate about the potentially harmful effects of overconsumption of isoflavone-intensive soy products. Soy is popular as a phytooestrogen for the same reason that it poses a danger to the thyroid: in large enough quantities it functions as a hormone and anti-thyroid agent. The isoflavones in soy belong to the *flavonoid* chemical family, and flavonoids are considered endocrine disruptors – plants that act as hormones, disrupting the endocrine system. Flavonoids typically act against the thyroid by inhibiting thyroid peroxidase (TPO), which disturbs proper thyroid function.

There are concerns for adult consumption of soy products. One UK study involving premenopausal women gave the subjects 60 grams of soy protein per day for a month. This was found to disrupt the menstrual cycle, with the effects of the isoflavones continuing for a full 3 months after stopping the soy in the diet. Another study found that intake of soy over a long period causes enlargement of the thyroid and suppresses thyroid function.

Isoflavones are also known to negatively affect fertility and sex hormones, and can have serious health effects in a number of mammals, including infertility, thyroid disease and liver disease.

In a February 18, 1999, official letter of protest to the Food and Drug Administration, Doerge and Daniel Sheehan, who at that time were the FDA's two key experts on soy, protested the health claims approved by the FDA on soy products, saying,

> There is abundant evidence that some of the isoflavones found in soy, including genistein and equol, demonstrate toxicity in estrogen-sensitive tissues and in the thyroid. This is true for a number of species, including humans. Additionally, isoflavones are inhibitors of the thyroid peroxidase, which makes T3 and T4. Inhibition can be expected to generate thyroid abnormalities, including goitre and autoimmune thyroiditis. There exists a significant body of animal data that demonstrates goitrogenic and even carcinogenic effects of soy products. Moreover, there are significant reports of goitrogenic effects from soy consumption in human infants and adults.

If you don't have a thyroid, soy is not something you need to worry about. But if you still have a thyroid, be careful about using too much soy. Tempeh, soy sauce and miso are far more easily digested and less likely to cause problems. Soy pills, powders and supplements, especially high-isoflavone supplements and daily overconsumption of soy foods, may all contribute to the worsening of your thyroid problem.

Coconut Oil/Medium-chain Triglycerides

If you search the topic 'thyroid' on the Internet or read some of the women's magazines, you'll find adverts touting coconut oil as a cure for thyroid disease and a weight-loss miracle food and supplement. Coconut oil is controversial, however.

Nutritionist Bruce Fife, author of *The Healing Miracles of Coconut Oil*, is a firm believer in coconut oil for thyroid patients. He says, 'Coconut oil by itself is not a thyroid cure. But when used as part of a thyroid-enhancing programme it can be invaluable in improving some forms of hypothyroidism and even bring about complete recovery.' Fife believes that coconut oil can rev up the metabolism, and he suggests replacing all refined vegetable oils with it, including margarine, shortening and hydrogenated oils. He also recommends using coconut products and foods such as coconut milk as much as possible in cooking.

Coconut oil contains medium-chain triglycerides (MCTs), which are a special type of saturated fat. It's theorized that MCTs may promote weight loss by increasing the burning of calories. Research conducted in Canada found that medium-chain fatty acids (MCFAs) such as those found in coconut oil are quickly oxidized in the liver, and this speed of oxidation leads to greater energy expenditure. No weight loss, however, was associated with the demonstrated increase in energy expenditure.

Research is contradictory. In one study, 66 women were put on a very low-carbohydrate diet for 4 weeks. Half received a regular fat supplement; the other half received an MCT supplement. Those on the MCT supplement had increased fat burning and less loss of muscle mass during the first 2 weeks, but these benefits declined during the last 2 weeks of the trial. Other trials showed that MCTs and coconut oil failed to enhance weight loss.

You can see if it works for you. And remember that the way to use coconut oil is *not* to add a few tablespoons to your diet on top of your regular foods, including fats. If you want to see if it's going to help, you need to cut out most of your other fats and oils and substitute coconut oil to see if you get any benefit.

PART 2

Metabolism, Weight Loss and the Thyroid

CHAPTER 3

Food and Metabolism

Make food a very incidental part of your life by
filling your life so full of meaningful things that
you'll hardly have time to think about food.

— PEACE PILGRIM

I have to admit that I went through numerous versions of this chapter. It started out as a 60-page dissertation on the entire process of digestion, nutrition, metabolism and the intricate hormonal interactions that affect appetite, fat-burning and blood sugar. When I realized that I was starting to talk medicalese – after all, do I need to use the term *gluconeogenesis* ten times in one chapter? – I knew it was time to go back to square one and answer the really important question: What are the key things about food, energy, metabolism and endocrinology that you need to know to help you lose weight? So if you want a comprehensive understanding of the whole physiology, I'd suggest a textbook on nutrition or endocrinology, where you can learn the details about gluconeogenesis (including how to pronounce it!). In the meantime, here are the key points that you need to know.

HOW FOOD BECOMES ENERGY

To understand how to lose weight, you first have to understand how food becomes energy in your body. Food is converted into energy by the processes of digestion and metabolism. Let's use lunch as an example: a turkey sandwich on white bread with mayonnaise, sweetened soda and a spinach salad. Where you see typical components – bread, turkey, mayonnaise, soda, spinach – your body sees carbohydrates (bread, spinach and soda), protein (turkey) and fat (mayonnaise). Each type of food is digested and metabolized into energy in different ways.

Digestion starts in the mouth, where the act of chewing, along with your saliva, which contains enzymes that start to break down food, work together to moisten and start dissolving food. The food heads down the oesophagus into your stomach, where enzymes and acids are released from the stomach lining. The food is chemically broken down, with each type of food headed for a different objective.

- **Carbohydrates such as fruits, vegetables, grains and sugars become sugar, or glucose, the energy source for cells.**
- **Proteins such as meat, poultry and dairy products become amino acids.**
- **Fats, such as those found in oils, nuts, fats, meat and dairy products, become triglycerides and fatty acids.**

Not all foods are digested at the same rate. Carbohydrates (which are not just starches but actually include everything from bread, rice and sugar to potatoes, green vegetables and fruits) are usually digested more quickly than proteins or fats. But how quickly you digest carbohydrates also depends on the type of carbohydrate. For example:

- **The sugars in simple carbohydrates in liquid form, such as in a sweetened soft drink, are already so small that they require almost no digestion before they can be absorbed into the stomach lining. Their small size enables them to pass quickly – usually in less than 30 minutes – into the small intestines, then the blood.**
- **Plain white bread is another refined, simple carbohydrate that has little to no fibre. With its easily dissolvable molecules, it will digest fairly**

quickly. (Contrast this with high-fibre bread, for example, which is less easily broken down and therefore is digested more slowly.)

- The carbohydrate that will be digested most slowly is the spinach, because, like all fruits and vegetables, it is a complex unrefined carbohydrate (meaning that it has to go through more digestive processes, which take longer, before it becomes glucose). The fibre in the spinach also slows down its digestion.
- The turkey and mayonnaise will require more time to digest because it takes longer for protein and fat to go through the first round of digestion by the stomach enzymes. Proteins and fats are more complicated molecules than carbohydrates and may take as long as 3½ hours to digest. This is why meals that contain sufficient protein and fat make you feel full longer.

After digestion in the stomach, food moves quickly through your small intestines, where all absorption of nutrients occurs.

- The carbohydrates in bread have been broken down into glucoses, which transfer easily across the lining (mucosa) of the small intestine into your blood.
- The indigestible carbohydrates in spinach, called fibre, move through your system unconverted into energy, since humans (unlike cows) do not have the enzymes to digest fibre.
- Turkey, partially digested by enzymes in the stomach, is met by more enzymes from your pancreas, helping to complete the breakdown of protein into amino acids.
- Once in the small intestine, the fat in mayonnaise is turned into a watery substance of fatty acids and cholesterols with the help of bile acids from the gallbladder. Inside the mucosa, fatty acids and cholesterols are rebuilt into fats called triglycerides and released into the blood.

Meanwhile, there is another process going on in your bloodstream! Glucose, amino acids and triglycerides start surging through the bloodstream to be used as energy, help in cellular repair, or stored as fat.

When faced with high amounts of glucose, your pancreas secretes a hormone known as insulin. Insulin's role is to keep blood glucose levels from rising too high. When insulin is present, glucose – your body's favourite and most easy-to-use energy source – is taken up by cells, especially the important area known as the mitochondria, sometimes called the powerhouse of the cell, since this is where the largest production of energy occurs.

What happens to the amino acids and triglycerides? Usually, triglyceride fats end up stored in fat tissue. They can be converted into glucose by your liver, but usually only as a last resort when glucose is not readily available, because it costs the body more energy to metabolize these stored fats into energy. In case of a brief starvation, the liver holds a 12-hour supply of glycogen, which it can convert into glucose to help fuel the body. Otherwise, the body is very stubborn about letting go of its fat and amino acid reserves. This is why it can be hard to lose weight, since the body will readily and quite efficiently use all the glucose it gets directly from food.

Once you have finished digesting all the carbohydrates you last ate, your liver will convert its stored glycogen back into glucose and release the glucose to help maintain blood sugar. When the liver runs out of glycogen, and in the absence of new carbohydrates or glucose sources, the liver shifts to a process called gluconeogenesis (there's that word!) and starts converting amino acids into glucose.

As you can see, your metabolism is going to do everything it can to:

- **make sure you get every glucose molecule out of the food you eat**
- **store sufficient fat so that you have energy sources during periods of 'starvation'.**

INSULIN

When you have eaten a concentration of simple carbohydrates – sweets and/or a fizzy drink, for example – the body generates a strong insulin response to prevent excess blood sugar. This large insulin response, in turn, can trigger a dramatic drop in blood sugar – sometimes to levels that are even too low – in the 3 to 5 hours after the simple carbohydrate was eaten. When blood glucose levels fall, an adrenaline surge can be triggered, which can then cause nervousness, anxiety, irritability and even palpitations. (This is the phenomenon observed in some children when they've had too much sugar.)

The same up-and-down pattern of insulin, glucose and adrenaline levels either doesn't happen at all or is severely blunted after eating a balanced meal that includes fats, proteins and fibre in addition to complex carbohydrates, because the processes of digestion and absorption are slowed down.

Higher blood glucose levels can occur for the following reasons:

- **consumption of too many carbohydrates, especially simple, refined carbohydrates**
- **eating too many calories, so excess calories are stored as fat, then released as glucose**
- **high stress levels that stimulate cortisol production**
- **other dysfunctions in the metabolic and hormonal systems.**

Insulin resistance can occur, in which the brain and some of the body's cells fail to react to the presence of insulin in the bloodstream.

This condition is not as severe as diabetes, where the cells cannot secrete enough insulin to maintain safe blood sugar levels. Instead, insulin levels may actually be high, yet the pancreas continues to pump out even more insulin in an attempt to store the glucose left in the blood. But the cells cannot react to the insulin that is released, and the glucose continues to circulate in the bloodstream. When you eat, glucose levels rise even higher. After a few years, the overworked pancreas begins to tire and may lose its ability to produce any insulin at all, leading to Type II diabetes. Insulin resistance is, in fact, sometimes called *prediabetes*.

The high levels of insulin circulating through the bloodstream also stimulate the storage of fat and amino acids and prevent the breakdown of fat and protein. They also prevent the release of glucagons.

The fat cells in your abdomen are particularly sensitive to high insulin levels and are very effective at storing energy – far more so than fat cells you'd find in other areas such as the lower body (i.e. hips, rear end, thighs). Because abdominal fat cells are so close to your digestive organs and there is an extensive network of blood vessels circulating in the abdominal area, it's even easier for fat cells to store excess glucose there.

Before it has progressed to full-scale Type II diabetes, insulin resistance is a reversible condition. Exercise, a reduction in simple carbohydrates and a reduction in calories can all help to reduce insulin levels. Exercise helps cells respond more effectively to insulin, which then helps reduce the excess glucose in the bloodstream before it is stored as fat. Fewer simple carbohydrates reduce the overall circulating blood glucose levels. And avoiding overeating prevents excess calories from all sources from being released into the bloodstream as glucose. The less glucose, the less insulin; when insulin levels are low, the body turns to fat reserves for energy and starts to break down large fat molecules into fatty acids for easy energy production.

Metabolic Syndrome

Taking insulin resistance a step further results in metabolic syndrome (also sometimes known as Syndrome X). Metabolic syndrome is usually characterized by insulin resistance plus elevated levels of cholesterol and triglycerides, as well as obesity.

The official diagnostic criteria for metabolic syndrome include:

- obesity, with a body mass index (BMI) greater than or equal to 25
- abdominal obesity (waist circumference greater than 40 inches in men and 35 inches in women)
- triglyceride levels above 150 mg/dL
- low HDL (high-density lipoprotein) cholesterol levels (less than 40 mg/dL in men and 50 mg/dL in women)
- high blood pressure (greater than or equal to 130/85 mm Hg)
- a high fasting glucose level, with fasting blood sugar more than 110 mg/dL.

Some experts estimate that as many as 1 in 4 adults have metabolic syndrome. These numbers are expected to rise as the population ages.

OTHER PLAYERS IN THE PROCESS
Glucagon

As I mentioned, in the presence of glucose your pancreas releases insulin. But if your blood sugar is low – for example, if you haven't eaten in 4 or 5 hours – the pancreas will secrete *glucagon*. It's like the opposite of insulin. Glucagon pulls sugars out of storage, first from the liver, then by converting fatty tissue back into glucose.

The higher the carbohydrate content of your last meal, the more insulin is produced and the less glucagon your body secretes. This pushes your body towards storing fat. Besides lower blood glucose levels, two other conditions are known to trigger the release of glucagon:

1. **Elevated blood levels of amino acids** – for example, after you eat a protein-heavy meal.
2. **Exercise** – whether the exercise itself or the drop in blood glucose stimulates the glucagon is not known, but there is definitely a relationship.

Leptin

Entering into the whole metabolism equation is the issue of leptin, a hormone produced by your fat cells that controls your body's fat-storage responses. When leptin is released by your fat cells, it is communicating to your brain how much fat you have stored. Enough leptin being released to the brain tells the brain – specifically your hypothalamus gland – there is enough fat stored now to avoid starvation, so you can stop eating. The 'stop eating' message is translated into a reduction in appetite and a speeding up in metabolism/energy expenditure.

When the body faces real starvation or perceived starvation such as a dramatic calorie reduction, leptin release is slowed or stopped. Lowered leptin levels communicate to the brain that there is insufficient fat stored to prevent possible starvation and food intake should be increased. Appetite will rise. This is the mechanism that makes you feel hungry when you go on a particularly low-calorie diet.

Logic would dictate that giving obese people leptin might help with weight loss, but in a rush to create leptin-based drugs this theory was tested and shown to be faulty. Interestingly, obese people tend to have very high levels of leptin. The real problem appears to be that, in people who are overweight, it's not a shortage of leptin that causes difficulties; it's that the brain is not getting the message. In essence, the brain is leptin resistant, meaning that the brain and metabolism think the body is starving even while the person is eating too much food.

If the brain isn't getting the right message about leptin in the first place, the metabolic circuit becomes broken. The brain cannot tell the body that enough fat is stored, food intake can slow down and energy expenditure can rise. More fat will accumulate and metabolism will slow down further.

Ghrelin

Ghrelin, sometimes referred to as the hunger hormone, is a hormone produced by your stomach that says 'it's time to eat now!' Ghrelin rises sharply before you eat and falls quickly afterward. The ghrelin signal itself has a short-term effect, lasting up to an hour. If you don't eat when the signal presents itself, it will go away fairly quickly and appetite will disappear.

When you lose weight, however, baseline ghrelin levels can go up. One study found ghrelin levels rose an average of 24 per cent in people on a slimming diet. In this way, it's thought that ghrelin may be part of the body's efforts to avoid starvation and maintain a particular weight range.

Adrenal Hormones: Cortisol and Adrenaline

Your hypothalamus, via the pituitary gland, directs the adrenal glands to secrete the hormones cortisol and adrenaline. Cortisol is released as part of your daily hormonal cycle, but both hormones can also be released in reaction to perceived stress – both physical and emotional – as part of the body's fight-or-flight response that is essential for survival. Adrenaline makes you energetic and alert, and increases metabolism. It also helps fat cells to release energy. Cortisol helps your body become even more effective at producing glucose from proteins and is designed to help quickly increase the body's energy in times of stress.

The problem is that many of us are under a constant state of stress for various reasons. This leads to a constant state of excess cortisol production. Excess cortisol stimulates glucose production. This excess glucose then typically is converted into fat, ending up as stored fat. There are many research studies showing that high levels of circulating cortisol increase the risk of obesity and increased fat storage – particularly abdominal obesity, which is one of the most dangerous types of obesity.

And excess adrenaline production means that the fat cells can become resistant to the effects of adrenaline. Eventually, the fat cells become unresponsive to adrenal stimulation to release fat, but through the presence of high cortisol they're more responsive to fat storage.

INFLAMMATION

The role of inflammation in metabolism and weight issues is just beginning to be studied. Usually, inflammation is a sign that your immune system is fighting off some sort of infection or attempting to heal an injury. So, for example, when your nasal passages swell during a respiratory infection, your immune system is sending white blood cells and other substances to help fight off germs, viruses and bacteria to reduce infection.

Some kinds of inflammation, however, are signs that the body is in a state of imbalance. For example, when you regularly eat foods to which you are allergic or sensitive, you can inflame the muscosal lining of your intestines. Eventually, the lining can become less and less able to prevent passage of larger molecules, and large molecules can pass into your bloodstream, a condition known as *leaky gut syndrome*. This condition has a connection to the development of various forms of autoimmune disease, including thyroid disease, as well as other conditions.

Researchers are now looking at the role of chronic inflammation in weight gain. One study in the *Journal of the American Medical Association* found that a particular inflammatory marker known as C-reactive protein (CRP) was increased by more than 50 per cent in obese women whose fat concentration centred mainly on their hips and thighs (i.e. pear-shaped distribution) and was increased by more than 400 per cent in obese women whose fat was centred on the waist and abdomen (i.e. apple-shaped distribution).

Interestingly, there are some studies that show exercise can actually reduce levels of inflammatory proteins. Antioxidants in fruits and vegetables also appear to help reduce pro-inflammatory hormones. And sufficient levels of omega-3 fats (found primarily in fatty fish and flaxseeds) and proper balance with omega-6 fats (found in common vegetable oils like corn, safflower and sunflower oil) appear to reduce inflammation as well.

METABOLISM

Now that you know about the process by which food is converted into energy and some of the various hormones and processes involved, it's time to look at the factors that affect the efficiency of that process. Metabolism actually refers to the way – not the speed – in which your body processes and uses the food you eat each day. The idea of a faster or slower metabolism is not really as accurate as the idea of an efficient, dysfunctional, or inefficient metabolism.

Metabolism itself is made up of several components:

- **Basal metabolism** – from 60 to 65 per cent of calories you eat each day are spent just keeping you alive and giving you energy for basic life support. If you were to lay in bed all day, you would still need a substantial number of calories to support basic body functions.
- **Physical activity** – 25 per cent of your calories go to movement and physical activity.
- **Thermic effect of food** – about 10 per cent of calories are spent processing the food you eat. For example, if you are eating 2,000 calories a day, 10 per cent of 2,000 is 200, so optimally you would be burning 200 calories a day simply eating and digesting your food.

The essential formula is that input should equal output.

INPUT	OUTPUT
Calories from food =	Calories expended from basal metabolism + Calories expended by activity + Calories expended digesting food (thermic effect)

Many overweight people do not eat any more than people of average weight. So it's clear that the problem for many must be on the output side of the equation. In most overweight people, either basal metabolism is lower, activity is less and/or the thermic effect of food is blunted. Bottom line: overweight people just don't burn as many calories as people of normal weight.

METABOLIC EFFICIENCY

The efficiency of your metabolism is affected by a number of factors.

Body Composition/Muscle Versus Fat

Muscle cells are as much as eight times more metabolically active than fat cells. So the greater the proportion of muscle to fat, the more efficient your metabolism is at burning fat. Ric Rooney and Bart Hanks of the Physique Transformation website say that a pound of muscle costs up to 50 calories a day to maintain; a pound of fat costs just 2. One study actually found that lifting weights boosted the resting metabolic rate by 9 per cent over 18 weeks by adding 4 pounds of muscle mass. By the time 2 pounds of muscle is gained – usually over 3 months or so – your extra muscle can burn as much as an extra 65 calories a day.

The amount of weight-bearing exercise you do has an effect on your metabolism. Building muscle mass usually requires some sort of weight-bearing or resistance work such as lifting weights, using exercise bands or hand weights, and other similar forms of exercise.

Brown Fat

According to Stephen Langer, an expert on weight loss and thyroid function, one lesser-known aspect of metabolism is brown fat, also known as brown adipose tissue (BAT). BAT is a special kind of adipose fat that collects below the neck and extends down the back. It helps convert deposits of body fat into heat. The hypothalamus helps your nervous system trigger the action of brown fat, whose specialized mitochondria are particularly effective at generating heat and energy. People who are overweight may have lost the assistance of brown fat, and their excess calories go into fat storage.

Aerobic Exercise

Aerobic exercise, which increases heart rate, will also raise metabolism while you're exercising. And some experts believe that aerobic exercise boosts your resting metabolism for several hours afterward, as your muscles burn calories to recover and repair themselves.

Food Intake

Metabolism is affected by how much you eat. When you are eating an insufficient amount of calories, your body perceives itself to be in starvation mode and will start to cannibalize your own muscle, burning it off for fuel. It will hold on to fat as protection. In his book *Turn Up the Heat*, Philip L Goglia talks about the impact of a too-low-calorie diet on weight problems:

> I have found that most of the people who come to me with weight and health problems are usually *already* ingesting *far fewer calories* than they should in order to efficiently fuel their bodies. Therefore, their metabolism, the body's calorie-burning furnace, is already running 25 to 60 per cent below its ideal metabolic-efficiency level. In turn, the body is storing much of the limited amounts of food these individuals eat as fat and wasting muscle tissue as an adaptive mechanism to create an alternative energy source.

At the same time, eating more food increases metabolism. One study found that as calorie intake increases, there is a corresponding increase in metabolic efficiency that is designed to maintain you around a particular body weight. However, if your caloric intake exceeds your body's ability to burn up those calories over time, the excess calories are converted into fat and glucose.

The Type of Food You Eat

Protein requires more energy to be broken down, digested and absorbed, and resting metabolic rate typically goes up after eating protein as much as two to three times more than after eating carbohydrates and fats.

Your Age

The body typically starts to lose muscle after age 30, so everything else being equal – activity level, calorie intake – you'll gain weight because of this loss of muscle.

Genetics

Some people simply have a naturally more efficient metabolism than others.

Nutritional Status

Metabolism requires the smooth running of many complex physiological processes. When there are nutritional deficiencies, particularly in antioxidant vitamins such as B and C, metabolism can become less efficient.

Water Intake/Hydration

When the body has taken in sufficient water, body temperature can be maintained for optimal metabolism. Dehydration can make the body temperature drop slightly, and with a reduction in temperature the body will attempt to help raise temperature by storing fat to act as an insulator. So drinking too little water can contribute to an inefficient metabolism and hoarding of fat.

Menopausal Status

The menopause also adds additional hormonal burdens to metabolism and weight loss. During the menopause, women become more effective at storing fat and less able to burn fat. After the menopause, an enzyme called adipose tissue lipoprotein lipase (AT-LPL) is more active. AT-LPL breaks fat down so that fat cells can absorb it. One study found that the burning ability of fat taken from the buttocks of postmenopausal women was 75 per cent less than in perimenopausal women.

Summary

As you can see, the body is a calorie miser, and there are a number of places that these complicated processes can fail, making it easier for you, especially as a thyroid patient, to gain weight, and making it harder to lose weight.

- You may be deficient in digestive enzymes.
- You may be eating too many starchy carbohydrates or too many carbs overall.
- You may be eating too few or too many calories.
- You may be eating too little protein or fat.
- Your blood sugar may be too high.
- You may be getting insufficient exercise and may have insufficient muscle.
- Your leptin may be imbalanced or you may be leptin resistant.
- Your adrenal system may be imbalanced due to stress.
- You may be insulin resistant or have metabolic syndrome.
- You may have a slower basal metabolism for any number of reasons.
- You may be burning fewer calories because you have less physical activity.
- You may have a blunted thermic effect of food.

The next chapter expands upon this understanding to explore the links between your thyroid, metabolism and weight-loss efforts.

CHAPTER 4

How Thyroid Dysfunction Affects Metabolism and Weight

Pain is inevitable, suffering is optional.

– M. KATHLEEN CASEY

You may think that if you have an undiagnosed thyroid condition, your weight problems will be over after it is treated. Unfortunately, that happy ending is for the minority of patients. The majority of thyroid patients struggle with a variety of symptoms, including fatigue, mood swings and, of course, weight gain or difficulty losing weight.

This is where the issue becomes particularly challenging, because there is a fear among some doctors even to connect thyroid and weight problems. Perhaps this is because, in the past, just as amphetamines were abused by doctors and patients for weight loss, thyroid drugs were also misused in a similar way. Doctors who were known to dispense amphetamines and thyroid drugs for weight loss – the 'diet doctors' – had a bad reputation. In fact, the stigma was so bad that today's medical specialists in weight loss call themselves 'bariatrics physicians', and they are more likely to be handing out antidepressants and suggesting gastric bypass than testing for an underactive thyroid.

Today's doctors are afraid that if they connect your weight with your thyroid, you may become a drug-seeker, looking for drugs inappropriately – in this case, looking to get thyroid drugs or taking too many thyroid drugs as a way to lose weight. They fear being lumped into the old category of the diet doctors.

Another reason doctors don't want to connect thyroid disease with weight gain is that they simply don't understand very much about nutrition, metabolism and the thyroid. They know the basic symptom list, they know how to do a thyroid-stimulating hormone (TSH) test, and they know how to write out prescriptions. But they don't know about nutrition. You've heard the old bromide about how most doctors spend about an hour on nutrition in medical school. Well, in addition to that hour, they spend a couple of hours on thyroid disease, and that completes their education on nutrition and metabolism. The complexities of the endocrine system, the delicate interplay that goes on between hormones, the brain, the stomach, the appetite and the ability to store and burn fat, are not topics most doctors have studied or even understand.

Most doctors really don't know what to do about losing weight. Doctors don't have much more advice than telling people to get off the couch, get more exercise and eat less. Even for those who don't have a thyroid problem, this advice obviously isn't working. And when you add in the difficulties of a thyroid problem, doctors have even less to offer.

What you will hear from endocrinologists, other doctors and even patients, however, are supposed 'facts' about thyroid disease and weight gain that are spread around without question, but should actually be looked at quite critically.

FACTS VERSUS MYTHS

There are a variety of myths about thyroid disease and weight gain. Here are the facts.

1. If You are Hyperthyroid, You May Not Lose Weight

Actually, a percentage of people who are actively hyperthyroid *gain* weight. Why they do is not clear. It may be they are simply so hungry that they are taking in more calories than even their revved-up metabolism can burn. Or it may be that their impaired endocrine system sets into motion a variety of the problems discussed in the last chapter, such as poor digestion, insulin resistance and adrenaline resistance.

2. If You are Hypothyroid, You May Not Gain Weight

There are in fact a small percentage of hypothyroid patients who have diffi-culty gaining weight, or who maintain a normal weight throughout diagno-sis and treatment. Also, some hypothyroid people do not have weight gain straight away, but find that over time it slowly creeps up on them.

3. If You are Hypothyroid, Your Weight Gain May be Significant

If you talk to some doctors, they will suggest to you that hypothyroidism can't cause more than a few pounds of weight gain. Not true. Just ask the thousands upon thousands of thyroid patients who were at perfectly normal weights – myself included – until they started to pile on weight faster than seemingly physically possible, only to get diagnosed with hypothyroidism shortly afterwards. Of course, there are always some patients who gain only a few pounds and who lose them fairly easily once treated, but they appear to be in the minority.

Laura, an active 51-year-old mother of two children, knew something was wrong when she started to gain weight and feel tired, moody and achy:

> I went from a vibrant, in-shape woman to a totally out-of-control, overweight couch potato! I wanted to scream but could not, since I also lost my voice! I did not want to leave my house and was too tired to do anything. I felt so sick I thought I would die! I gained about 40 pounds [2 st 12] in a period of about 3 months. That alone was pretty scary.

Elizabeth is 61 and describes herself as at least 70 pounds (5 stone) over-weight. In the past, the heaviest she had been was 190 (13 st 8) after two pregnancies.

> In 1999, I was told I had nodes on my thyroid and had a biopsy, which showed all was well. I had a severe case of vertigo in 2000 and the doctor I was taken to found out that my heart rate was out of control and my thyroid readings were bad. I was seriously hyperthyroid. Diagnosis: multitoxic nodular

thyroid. I went to an endocrinologist and he had me take RAI (a high dose) and then I was put on thyroid medication. He never told me that I was going to gain this much weight. I ballooned up to 230 pounds [16 st 6]. That is my current weight! So I went from 190 to 230! What I find most frightening is the way my body has changed shape. Also my neck, which used to be long and graceful, is now squat, short and I have these fat bulges in the indentations of my collarbones. I kept crying to the endocrinologist about how big I was getting. He said nothing and did nothing. I then went to a woman endocrinologist – she looked at me and pooh-poohed everything I said. She said I was fat from eating! At this point my regular internist takes care of me. But I must say that not a day goes by that I do not cry in the privacy of my home. I am so heavy my back is killing me. I barely have enough breath or energy to do things like I used to. It seems the doctors are unwilling to see the pain we are in. In plain English, I am not the same person I was before I had RAI. I am so miserably unhappy. I must try to get a grip on my weight before it does me in altogether.

4. If You Are Treated with Radioactive Iodine (RAI), You Will Most Likely Become Hypothyroid and You Will in All Likelihood Gain Weight

Doctors who tell you that they can somehow calculate just the right amount of RAI are living in fantasyland, because most patients post-RAI become hypothyroid, and many complain of weight gain. In fact, one research study found that more than 85 per cent of patients receiving RAI became hypothyroid and, despite being treated with medication, their median weight gain was 11 pounds after 6 months, 20 pounds after 12 months, and 25 pounds after 2 years. Before the therapy, 27.5 per cent were considered underweight by body mass index calculations, and 19.3 per cent were obese, with a body mass index above 30. Two years after treatment, only 8.7 per cent of patients were underweight, and 51.3 per cent were obese. Overall, the researchers found that there was a 32 per cent increase in obesity in previously hyperthyroid patients following RAI therapy, with the main weight gain coming in the first 2 years.

Miya had this experience:

> I used to be chronically underweight. In high school I wore a size 6 and I'm 5'9"! My mom was convinced I had an eating disorder. I always felt light-headed and would get dizzy spells. When my thyroid was hyper, I was literally eating four to seven meals a day. I ate Dairy Queen [ice cream] on a regular basis and was out-eating my 6'2" boyfriend. I gained maybe 5 pounds the whole time (months and months) I was hyper. Once I went on medication I started to gain. I guess I began to be a weight that my body was supposed to be. I went up to a size 10, then a 12. When I was diagnosed, I was about 130 pounds [9 st 4]. When I had RAI, after a year of Tapazole, I think I was about 150 [10 st 10]. After RAI, there was a two-week period where I literally gained 10 or 15 pounds. It was insane. My weight went up to 175 [12½ stone].

5. Thyroid Cancer Patients Can Have Weight Problems

Some doctors will suggest that thyroid cancer, either in its early stages or after treatment, doesn't cause weight problems. Not true.

Jody was diagnosed with thyroid cancer at age 21 and had a complete thyroidectomy followed by one radiation treatment:

> During the time period that my thyroid was all out of whack when I was going through all the ultrasounds and biopsies to determine cancer or not, I gained 40 pounds. Yes, I went from a very healthy and in-shape size 6 to a tired, miserable and flabby size 16. I hated what had happened to my body as well as my mental well-being. I felt disgusting and that I had lost control of the one thing that I used to be very in control of. After the surgery, I could only thank God for getting me through it all and I could call myself a cancer survivor.

6. If All or Part of Your Thyroid is Removed, You Can Still Gain Weight

But it's not guaranteed that you'll gain weight in this situation, because total thyroidectomy is most often done for thyroid cancer patients. And if you've had thyroid cancer, doctors do not typically wait until you become hypothyroid and your TSH levels elevate before they start thyroid hormone replacement. It's usually started straight away, and levels of thyroid hormone replacement are high enough to suppress thyroid hormone production, which means that you will be kept at a hyperthyroid or nearly undetectable TSH level. Still, even with a TSH at a hyperthyroid level, you may find weight piling on or impossible to lose.

7. The Weight Will Probably Not Just Melt Off After You Start Thyroid Hormone Replacement

There is always the story of the thyroid patient who started taking his or her medication or natural thyroid and lost 20 pounds in a month. But these accounts are few and far between. More likely is the loss of a few pounds, usually water weight, as the water retention of hypothyroidism starts to abate, then ... nothing. The scales come to a grinding halt.

CHALLENGES TO WEIGHT LOSS FOR THYROID PATIENTS

Even if your thyroid treatment is optimized, as described in Chapter 2, as a thyroid patient you may still face a variety of challenges that make it more difficult to lose weight than it is for the typical person. I've focused primarily on hypothyroidism because the end result for almost all thyroid conditions is a surgically removed, radioactively ablated, or otherwise underactive or non-functioning thyroid – or hypothyroidism.

Diagnosis Delay

For many people who become hypothyroid, it can be months or even years from the time their thyroid condition develops to when it is diagnosed and treated. During this period, a variety of symptoms can appear, even before

TSH elevates enough to officially qualify for a conventional diagnosis of hypothyroidism. Even slight decreases in metabolism mean fewer calories burned every day, so even if you ate the same amount and kept up your same level of activity over time, you would see weight gain due to the slight reduction in metabolism. Unfortunately, many people who are becoming hypothyroid also experience fatigue, low energy and muscle pain, which makes them less likely to exercise. So you have another factor that can further reduce metabolism. Finally, as you become more tired, you may eat more to unconsciously try to generate energy. So it's a triple whammy to your metabolism: you're eating more food, burning off even less of it because of a lowered basal resting metabolism, and doing less physical activity.

If this resulted in a metabolism that was 350 calories a day less efficient, you could gain a pound or more every 10 days, or 3 pounds a month. Go undiagnosed for a year and that's 36 pounds. It can be even more, because the more weight you gain, the more efficient your body becomes at fat storage and the less active you typically become. All the more reason to become your own best advocate and push for diagnosis and treatment as early as possible.

Hyperthyroidism

As hyperthyroidism develops, some people actually enjoy the ability to eat anything they want without weight gain or even with weight loss. Excess energy in some hyperthyroid people also results in their doing a great deal of exercise. So during this period, there's an increase in resting metabolism and often an increase in activity level that often outweighs increased appetite. Or, if appetite remains the same, some people enjoy desirable weight loss that occurs as they eat normal amounts but lose weight because of improved metabolic efficiency.

The problem is that hyperthyroidism needs to be treated. It can cause rapid pulse and high blood pressure, and untreated hyperthyroidism puts you at risk of *thyroid storm*, an episode of uncontrollably high blood pressure and heart rate that can result in heart attack or stroke. So at a minimum, your doctor will give you anti-thyroid drugs and perhaps beta blockers, to help slow things down temporarily and see if you respond. Or you may get RAI treatment that permanently makes you hypothyroid.

The problem is that you may continue to eat as you did before. If you were eating at higher-calorie levels and all of a sudden you go on anti-thyroid drugs to slow down your thyroid, and beta blockers to slow down your heart rate, it's like taking your metabolism from 60 to 0. You're going to be burning up fewer calories, and you can start gaining weight quickly on your former calorie level. The double whammy comes when you find yourself feeling tired, so you cut back on activity and burn even fewer calories.

Even if you did not increase your food intake, you may have been eating at a level that maintained your weight. But after your diagnosis, and after your metabolism adjusts to anti-thyroid medication and beta blockers, you may find yourself gaining weight if you don't cut calories and/or increase physical activity.

Erich was a cross-country runner, 5'10", who kept himself at a trim 145 pounds (10 st 5) for most of his life, until he developed hyperthyroidism, went on anti-thyroid drugs, then had a thyroidectomy:

> My weight just prior to surgery had climbed to an astounding 195 pounds [13 st 13], fully 30 pounds more than I'd weighed for the majority of my life. Following surgery, I was placed on a minimal dosage of medication, which failed to provide me with the necessary supplement for my removed thyroid gland. Gradually, the dosage was increased (sometimes by my taking two pills on my own) until the point where I was taking 500 mcg per day. Unfortunately, the higher dosage failed to alleviate many of the symptoms of hypothyroidism such as cold hands, lethargy, weight gain, etc. By the time I switched doctors, my weight had climbed to approximately 236 pounds [16 st 12].

Another problem for people who start out with hyperthyroidism is the delay in getting on thyroid hormone replacement after RAI. Honestly, I have no idea what motivates some of the doctors who are treating thyroid patients, but if you are hyperthyroid and going to have RAI, your doctor should sit down and tell you these things:

1. It's likely that you will become hypothyroid.
2. This can happen quickly, maybe several weeks after RAI, or it may take months.
3. Be aware of hypothyroidism symptoms. If you have any of these symptoms, make a doctor's appointment immediately so that your thyroid levels can be checked.
4. As soon as symptoms appear and/or you have an elevation in TSH above a certain level, you will need to start thyroid hormone replacement drugs.

Most of you will not have this discussion with your doctor. Unfortunately, the longer you go with your TSH elevating and without thyroid hormone replacement treatment, the more likely it is that you will gain excess weight.

Once you've had RAI, forget about being hyperthyroid and start considering yourself hypothyroid. Familiarize yourself with hypothyroidism symptoms and treatments (my book *Living Well with Hypothyroidism* can help), and take control of your own health. Monitor your symptoms. If you have to, push for proper treatment for your now-hypothyroid condition.

Digestion and Elimination

Many doctors don't tell you that thyroid disease causes water retention and bloating – especially hypothyroidism, which can cause puffiness and bloating in the face, eye area, arms, hands, legs and feet. You also may not know that the body will hold on to water fiercely, unless you are getting enough water. Because you feel or look bloated or swollen, you may not drink enough water, but that is counterproductive. Dehydration can interfere with proper metabolism.

Hypothyroidism also slows down digestion and elimination. In fact, constipation is one of the most common symptoms, even for people who are treated. Slower and less efficient digestion and elimination means that toxins spend more time in the intestines, where they can do damage and pass into your body. Allergens spend more time in contact with your intestinal lining, where they can cause irritation and inflammation. All of these factors can impede weight loss.

Autoimmune Disease

Most thyroid disease is due to autoimmune conditions, like Hashimoto's disease and Graves' disease. Autoimmune diseases are conditions where there is internal inflammation. And, as noted in the previous chapter, inflammation can be a factor that impedes weight loss.

Endocrine Imbalances

The thyroid is part of the endocrine system. The endocrine system releases hormones and its key players include:

- pituitary gland/hypothalamus
- pineal gland
- thyroid gland
- parathyroid glands
- thymus gland
- adrenal glands
- pancreas
- ovaries
- testes
- gastrointestinal system.

The endocrine system is very much geared towards balance, and an imbalance in one area seems to set into motion a cascade of other imbalances in many people. Among these, the underlying endocrine dysfunction of a thyroid problem means that you face a higher risk of other endocrine imbalances and conditions, including:

- insulin resistance
- metabolic syndrome/syndrome X
- type II diabetes
- adrenaline resistance
- adrenal exhaustion
- leptin resistance
- deficiencies or imbalances in oestrogen, progesterone, testosterone and dehydroepiandrosterone (DHEA).

All of the above factors can interfere with weight loss.

Some thyroid patients also overuse caffeine and herbal stimulants for weight loss and energy, which further stimulates and aggravates the adrenal glands and contributes to worsening adrenal exhaustion.

Body Temperature

The reduction in body temperature associated with an underactive or inactive thyroid can communicate to your brain that you are facing a period of starvation. This sends out a variety of signals that increase appetite, encourage fat storage and discourage fat-burning – all as a means of ensuring survival.

Metabolism

The slowdown in metabolism may be communicating to your brain that you are facing a period of starvation, therefore increasing appetite, encouraging fat storage and discouraging fat-burning as a way to ensure your survival. Overall, a lower basal resting metabolism means that you either need to eat less or have higher physical activity, in order to prevent excess calorie intake and weight gain.

Another aspect of metabolism that is affected by hypothyroidism is the ability of cells to use oxygen, which is impaired in some people with thyroid dysfunction. This reduced oxygen utilization makes cells less effective at converting food into energy – another factor that encourages fat storage.

Starvation Dieting

Many thyroid patients have already gone to extremely low-calorie starvation diets in attempts to lose weight. This sort of diet wreaks havoc on the metabolism, making it think that you are facing starvation and turning on a whole host of appetite-increasing, fat-storing hormones, slowing the metabolism in order to prevent possible starvation.

Exercise

When you have a thyroid dysfunction, even with optimal treatment you may feel more fatigued than normal. This level of fatigue may mean that you exercise less and move around less, which reduces the amount of energy you expend.

Thyroid disease also commonly causes joint and muscle aches and pains, carpal tunnel syndrome, tarsal tunnel syndrome and tendonitis, all of which make exercise and movement harder and may discourage you from exercising. Again, less exercise means you expend less energy.

In both cases, the less you exercise and the less physical activity, the more likely you are to lose muscle mass. And reduced muscle mass also reduces metabolism.

Fatigue and Food Intake

Many people with thyroid problems experience ongoing fatigue. When you are tired, one of the body's ways to try to generate energy is to increase your appetite, encouraging you to eat to get energy.

Carbohydrate Cravings

Dutch researchers studying the energy and nutrient intake of thyroid patients found that thyroid disease, and hyperthyroidism in particular, may be linked to increased appetite for carbohydrates. This increased craving for and intake of carbohydrates appears to stem from various changes in brain chemistry and sympathetic nervous system activity due to the thyroid condition.

Depression

Thyroid disease can trigger or worsen depression. Depression is known to trigger eating in some people, and especially increase carbohydrate cravings. It can also make you less likely to exercise and disrupt your ability to get restorative sleep.

Sleep Disruptions

Thyroid patients may have difficulty getting restorative sleep, which affects fat-burning, serotonin and hormone levels.

Allergies/Sensitivities

One of the known causes of thyroid problems is coeliac disease, or gluten intolerance and sensitivity. Thyroid disease seems to make people more likely to have food allergies and sensitivities (e.g. wheat, milk, cheese, eggs, soy and citrus allergies). As a thyroid patient, you are also at greater risk of candidiasis – yeast overgrowth – and the sensitivity or allergy to yeast can become an impediment to effective weight loss.

All of these allergies and sensitivities can cause inflammation and disrupted digestion, and ultimately leaky gut/dysbiosis, which can further interfere with weight-loss efforts.

PART 3

Key Weight-Loss Issues

CHAPTER 5

Blood Sugar, Hormones, Allergies and Toxins

It's a very odd thing –
As odd as can be –
That whatever Miss T. eats
Turns into Miss T.

– WALTER DE LA MARE

The endocrine system maintains a delicate balance in the body, and when there is a dysfunction in your thyroid it can set into motion a host of other imbalances, sensitivities and abnormalities that all contribute to weight-gain or weight-loss difficulties. This chapter looks at some of the challenges that are more common in thyroid patients.

BLOOD SUGAR IRREGULARITIES

One thing you should consider is getting your blood sugar tested. At a minimum, you can get a glucose level from a home test kit, but preferably get a fasting glucose and even a glucose tolerance test (GTT) to evaluate whether your blood sugar is low, normal, high-normal, or elevated. If it is high-normal or elevated, this can in part contribute to your difficulty losing weight, and it is also a sign that you are either becoming insulin resistant, are prediabetes, or already have Type II diabetes.

In addition to using the blood sugar-balancing herbs (such as Glucosol) discussed in Chapter 6, as well as following a low-glycaemic diet and an exercise programme, your practitioner may wish to give you antidiabetes medication such as metformin.

Metformin helps to regulate blood glucose levels by reducing the amount of glucose produced by the liver, limiting the amount of glucose absorbed from food, and helping insulin to work better to reduce the amount of glucose in the blood. One study found that metformin was associated with weight loss, better glycaemic control and enhanced insulin sensitivity of visceral fat, which is the deep fat surrounding organs. Another study found that insulin-resistant people given metformin had a 31 per cent less chance of developing diabetes than control subjects with insulin resistance. Metformin can help to reduce cholesterol and triglyceride levels, and does not cause low blood sugar levels as often as some other drugs in its class (like glipizide).

On the downside, metformin can have a number of unpleasant side-effects including diarrhoea, nausea and vomiting. The most common side-effect was diarrhoea, which occurred in 53 per cent of metformin-treated subjects involved in a double-blind clinical trial. Nausea/vomiting occurred in 26 per cent of subjects in the same trial. Other common side-effects included flatulence, loss of strength, indigestion, abdominal discomfort and headache. Less common side-effects include abnormal stools, low blood sugar, muscle pain, light-headedness, shortness of breath, nail disorders, rash, increased sweating, taste disorders, chest discomfort, chills, flu symptoms, flushing and heart palpitations. In very rare circumstances, metformin has caused *lactic acidosis*, which is a build-up of lactic acid in the cells and bloodstream; it is fatal in 50 per cent of cases. Symptoms of lactic acidosis are subtle at first and include muscle pain, lethargy, a sense of not feeling well, breathing problems, sleepiness, abdominal aches, nausea, vomiting and severe weakening of the muscles in the legs and arms.

Patients with kidney disease, a history of shock, heart attack, liver disease or septicaemia should not take metformin. Also, people with congestive heart failure, a known sensitivity to metformin, or metabolic acidosis should not take metformin. Excessive intake of alcohol must be avoided because it raises the risk of lactic acidosis.

ADRENAL IMBALANCES

There is a strong connection between
and the thyroid. A malfunctioning adrenal
efforts. At one end, being in a situation of ad
produce too much cortisol, which can contribu
constant release of adrenaline can cause resistance to it
less efficient. At the other end, a low-functioning adrenal
adrenal insufficiency, can slow down overall metabolism an
thyroid problems.

Adrenal fatigue often develops after periods of intense or lengthy
cal or emotional stress, when overstimulation of the glands finally lea
them unable to meet the body's needs. Some other names for this condition
include non-Addison's hypoadrenia, subclinical hypoadrenia, hypoadren-
alism and neurasthenia. Symptoms include:

- excessive fatigue and exhaustion
- non-refreshing sleep (you get sufficient hours of sleep but wake fatigued) or sleep disturbances
- feeling overwhelmed by or unable to cope with stressors
- feeling run-down
- craving salty and sweet foods
- feeling most energetic in the evening
- experiencing low stamina, slow to recover from exercise
- being slow to recover from injury, illness or stress
- having difficulty concentrating, brain fog
- poor digestion
- low immune function
- food or environmental allergies
- premenstrual syndrome or difficulties that develop during the menopause
- consistent low blood pressure
- extreme sensitivity to cold.

The adrenals produce hormones that help to balance blood sugar, which helps your body to manage daily ebbs and flows of energy. When blood sugar drops, the adrenals release hormones that cause the blood sugar to

es when you're
se from the days
ay, it kicks in for
k pressures. But
lands, and even-
hormones.

cannot diagnose
iagnose extreme
potentially fatal
, or Cushing's
c or complemen-
our adrenal func-

tips:

the function of the adrenal glands
ystem can sabotage weight-loss
renal stress means that you
e to weight gain, and a
making metabolism
land, also called
can worsen
physi-
es

othyroidism have found that low-dose hydrocortisone can help their immune system and can resolve many symptoms.

- Pantothenic acid, 100–500 mg with each meal, can promote proper adrenal balance.
- As much as you may want them, stimulants are the equivalent of accelerating too fast and flooding the engine of a car. It puts further stress on the adrenals to work harder and produce more energy, and ends up further depleting the adrenal glands. Things to avoid include caffeine, ephedra, guarana, kola nuts and prescription stimulants.

OTHER HORMONAL IMBALANCES AND DEFICIENCIES

Imbalances of progesterone and oestrogen – either too much or too little, or an improper ratio of one to the other – can slow down your digestion or make you more efficient at fat storage. Not enough melatonin, pregnenolone or DHEA can also interfere with weight loss.

But the answer is not to start self-treating with over-the-counter progesterone creams or to order oestradiol creams, nor to hit the healthfood shops for bottles of melatonin, pregnenolone or DHEA. Whether or not they require a prescription, these are all hormones, and hormones can have powerful effects and side-effects. So you need to have your levels tested and deficiencies and imbalances assessed before you start adding hormones to the mix. For a thyroid patient who is already taking a hormone supplement, it is particularly essential to find a practitioner who can work with you to help determine the best possible mix of supplements. It's an art and a science not particularly suited to our own amateur efforts at diagnosis and treatment.

Dr David Brownstein, author of *The Miracle of Natural Hormones*, believes that balancing the entire hormonal system may be a key to weight loss for some people:

> In order to achieve the best results, I feel it is necessary to balance out the entire hormonal system. This can include the use of the adrenal hormones (i.e. DHEA and pregnenolone), ovarian hormones (i.e. using natural progesterone and natural estrogens and natural testosterone), growth hormone, melatonin and others. I find using small amounts of each of these hormones in combination much more effective than using one hormone individually. Sometimes, patients need a combination of treatments to help them achieve their optimum health.

FOOD ALLERGIES AND SENSITIVITIES

Sensitivities or full-scale allergies to particular foods or pathogens can cause inflammation in your intestinal system, making weight loss difficult, if not impossible. Food sensitivities and intolerances are quite common, but full-scale food allergies are less so. One report found that while 1 in 3 people think they have a food allergy, only 1 in 50 actually have. An allergy is defined as a reaction to a food or substance that could potentially trigger a life-threatening response such as anaphalactic shock, airway swelling or difficulty breathing. A food sensitivity is more likely to cause migraine headaches, fatigue, bloating, skin rashes, or diarrhoea.

The most common allergenic foods include:

- wheat
- dairy foods
- corn
- soy
- fish (especially shellfish)
- nuts
- fruits.

I'm fairly allergic to tree fruits (apples, pears, cherries, peaches, plums) and certain nuts such as walnuts, pecans and cashews (but not the common allergen peanuts). I also have seasonal hay fever, and these fruit/nut allergies are apparently more common in people who have hay fever. Interestingly, applesauce and baked or canned fruits are fine for me, because the allergen is apparently destroyed by cooking.

Inflammation occurs when you have a food allergy or sensitivity. This sort of inflammation gradually wears away the ability of your intestinal surface to filter out pathogens and toxins. Eventually, like a window screen that has developed holes, bigger particles can pass through your stomach and intestinal lining directly into the bloodstream, which triggers inflammation and irritation, interfering with your body's ability to absorb nutrients.

If you suspect food sensitivities or allergies, you don't need to head off for expensive allergy testing. One of the primary ways to assess them is to try an elimination/rotation diet. Stop eating a particular food for about a week, then reintroduce it in a larger quantity. Keep track of any symptoms you have over the next several days including aches, pains, headache, fatigue, stomach upset, skin eruptions, itching, mood swings and other strong reactions.

If you're going to do an elimination test diet, start with some of the most common allergens for people with thyroid problems: wheat, dairy, corn, soy and fish. Check the ingredients list of supplements and processed foods to make sure you're avoiding all sources of the allergen being tested. Sometimes it seems as if flour, corn oil, hydrogenated soy derivatives and soy proteins are in everything from power bars to breakfast cereals.

You can also pursue more formalized testing with an integrative or functional medicine expert or an allergist. A specialized blood test known as enzyme-linked immunosorbent assay (ELISA) is considered a state-of-the-art way to diagnose food sensitivities.

Obviously, if you discover a food to which you have a sensitivity or allergy, one of the key things you can do is eliminate it from your diet, or at least cut back significantly on consumption of the food to see if it aids you in your weight-loss efforts and helps to alleviate other symptoms.

CANDIDIASIS

Thyroid patients seem to be more susceptible to candidiasis – a chronic overgrowth of the fungus *Candida* – also known as chronic yeast infection. The condition was brought to the public's attention by the late Dr William Crook in his 1983 book, *The Yeast Connection*, and is considered to be the cause of – or is more common in people with – many hard-to-diagnose chronic illnesses.

If you have been on long-term antibiotic therapy, have a diet high in sugars, have used steroids or have a suppressed immune system, you are at higher risk for developing candidiasis. There are a number of other risk factors. They are outlined at length in Dr Crook's several definitive books on the topic.

The symptoms of candidiasis are fairly wide-ranging and include:

- frequent vaginal and genital yeast infections, including 'jock itch'
- frequent oral yeast infections (thrush)
- frequent infections of the nipple/breast when breast-feeding
- chronic ear, upper respiratory, allergic or sinus problems
- urticaria (hives, wheals, or welts), itching or burning sensation in the skin
- stomach, digestive and elimination problems
- fluid retention, swelling and bloating
- skin problems
- difficulty losing weight, or inappropriate weight gain.

These are just a few of the dozens of other symptoms attributed to *Candida* overgrowth.

Detecting *Candida* involves one or more tests, including:

- Candida immune complex assay test – this is a blood test that can detect the presence of antibodies that fight off yeast infections.
- Stool test – an exam of stool under a microscope may reveal the presence of *Candida*.
- Candida culture – in the case of oral, genital, or nipple thrush, a culture can be taken and analysed.

Treating candidiasis can be a complex process and may require monitoring by a good nutritionally-orientated doctor or practitioner. Treatment is typically multifaceted and may include the following tactics.

Changes to Diet

Dietary changes depend on the severity of symptoms. Some of the most extreme *Candida* diets suggest eliminating the foods that 'feed' yeast, including anything with yeast itself (such as breads), plus sugar, flour, fruits, dairy, certain meats, mushrooms and fermented products like vinegars and alcoholic drinks. Other suggestions include eliminating only those foods that are particularly troublesome. (Again, Dr Crook's books cover the entire yeast issue and provide specific guidelines on the diets.)

Supplements

Anti-yeast supplements are sometimes recommended, including garlic, biotin, caprylic acid, pau d'arco and others that are thought to help combat yeast.

Probiotics

Probiotics are supplements that contain live bacteria – the 'good' bacteria found in fermented foods such as miso and dairy products such as yogurt and some cheeses – that we are meant to have in sufficient quantities in our intestinal system. One of the more well-known bacterium in this category is *acidophilus*, the live cultures found in yogurt. A Finnish study found that giving probiotic supplements to pregnant women close to delivery and then to their newborns could help prevent childhood allergies in the babies. Allergy experts say this is evidence that probiotic bacteria can train the immune system to resist allergic reactions, including candidiasis.

Anti-fungal Drugs

Prescription anti-fungal drugs may be necessary in order to eliminate the *Candida* infection completely. Some of the drugs your doctor can prescribe include:

- fluconazole (Diflucan)
- terbinafine hydrochloride (Lamisil)
- nystatin
- itraconazole (Sporanox).

COELIAC DISEASE/GLUTEN SENSITIVITY

Coeliac disease, also known as coeliac sprue, coeliac sprue-dermatitis or gluten intolerance, is a chronic disease of the digestive system that prevents absorption of nutrients from food. People who have coeliac disease have an allergic sensitivity to gluten, a protein that is found in grains such as wheat, rye, barley and possibly oats. Eating these foods causes damage to the mucosal lining of the intestine, which leads to an inability to digest and absorb nutrients properly.

Coeliac disease can first appear in infants when they begin to eat gluten products. However, it may not be diagnosed at that time, and symptoms flare and diminish through adolescence and into adulthood, when symptoms reappear again. Most cases are diagnosed in people in their 30s and 40s.

Symptoms of coeliac disease and gluten sensitivity include:

- diarrhoeal, watery, odorous stools
- abdominal bloating, cramps, excessive or explosive gas
- weight loss or gain
- failure to gain weight and growth retardation in infants and children
- weakness, fatigue, including muscle weakness
- bone pain
- tingling and numbness in hands and feet
- absence of menstrual periods, delayed start of menstrual periods in adolescents

- infertility in women and men
- impotence
- orthostatic hypotension, where blood pressure drops upon standing, after being in bed or sitting down, which can cause dizziness or fainting.

The main way to diagnose coeliac disease is with a blood test to measure circulating antibodies to gluten – antigliadin, antiendomysium and antireticulin. A finger-prick test that does an analysis known as an IgA tissue transglutaminase (tTG) auto-antibody assay can be done to help diagnose coeliac disease. In some cases, endoscopic examination of the small bowel or a biopsy is necessary to make a diagnosis.

Many adults spend years being misdiagnosed, and are commonly told they have irritable bowel syndrome, which is a far less serious condition not treated with a gluten-free diet. It's particularly important to get a diagnosis of coeliac disease as early as possible, because the more delayed the diagnosis, the more risky the disease can be.

People with coeliac disease must stay on a gluten-free diet for the rest of their lives or risk damaging their small intestine and further losing the ability to absorb nutrients. A gluten-free diet means total avoidance of all wheat, rye and barley, and products made from them. There is some disagreement as to whether oats are also to be avoided. Be careful to avoid hidden glutens such as vegetable protein and malt, modified food starch, some soy sauces and distilled vinegars, among other food items. A good support group can help you learn how to eat gluten-free among today's variety of food options. It's essential to stay on the gluten-free diet for life. One Italian study found that the death rate for those who failed to stick to a gluten-free diet was six times higher than for those adhering to the diet.

The incidence of coeliac disease in various autoimmune disorders is 10 to 30 times higher compared to the general population. Even a sensitivity to gluten (and not full coeliac disease) may contribute to the development of an autoimmune disease, so it's important to be aware of the connection. Some patients have found that, independent of any testing or diagnosis, they have been able to reduce symptoms and more effectively lose weight on a gluten-free diet.

PARASITES

There are a variety of parasitic infections ranging from microscopic parasites like *giardia, amoeba, cryptosporidium* and *blastocystishominis* to larger parasites such as various worms and parasitic insects. You can pick up these parasites from a variety of sources, including improperly cooked foods, water, poor sanitation or hygiene, travel to tropical climates, exposure to animals or their faeces, insect bites and other means.

The symptoms of various parasitic infections vary, but often include intestinal problems and can include difficulty losing weight. Diagnosis depends on the suspected parasite and may include a physical exam, stool samples, urine samples, blood tests, biopsies, ultrasound, x-ray and tape tests (applying tape around the anal region to examine for microscopic worms).

Treatments depend on the type of infection and can include anti-parasitic drugs, steroids, pain-relievers, anti-inflammatories, antihistamines and antibiotics for relief of symptoms or to treat various infections. Some herbal remedies are fig andrographis root, garlic, wormseed, turmeric and pumpkin seeds, among others. There are also a number of parasite-cleansing systems and herbal combination remedies available.

Parasites are a complex issue, so you should not self-diagnose or self-treat. If you suspect that you may have any risk factors or symptoms of parasites – and many of us don't realize how pervasive parasitic infections are – you should start by reading one of the definitive books on the topic, such as *Guess What Came to Dinner? Parasites and Your Health* by Ann Louise Gittleman, then consulting with a practitioner who can help you to diagnose and treat the infection.

COPPER/ZINC BALANCE

One overlooked but important consideration for thyroid patients is copper overload. Dr Gittleman, in another key book, *Why Am I Always So Tired?* explores this issue:

Copper and zinc tend to work in a seesaw relationship with each other in the body. When the levels of one of these minerals rise in the blood and tissues, the levels of its counterpart tend to fall. Ideally, copper and zinc should be in a 1:8 ratio in favour of zinc in the tissues. But stress, overexposure to copper, or a low intake of zinc can throw the critical copper-zinc balance off, upsetting normal body functioning.

Gittleman believes that a copper-zinc imbalance can slow weight loss and impede conversion of T4 to T3, even in people whose thyroid hormone levels are normal.

To determine whether you have excess copper or a copper-zinc imbalance, you should have your practitioner run a trace elements analysis. This test uses a small hair sample to assess your nutritional levels of various minerals and metals.

Gittleman recommends that if you are found to have high copper levels, you should avoid foods that have high copper levels, including soy products, yeast, wheat bran/wheat germ, chocolate, mushrooms, nuts, seeds (except pumpkin), shellfish, organ meats and tea. She also recommends avoiding foods and drinks that deplete zinc, including alcohol, coffee, sugar and excessive carbohydrates, while emphasizing zinc-rich foods such as eggs, chicken, turkey, red meats, game and pumpkin seeds. Gittleman's book includes specific guidelines on copper-zinc balances.

CHAPTER 6

Drugs, Supplements and Herbs

I don't waste time thinking, 'Am I doing it right?'
I ask, 'Am I doing it?'

– GEORGETTE MOSBACHER

Drugs and supplements can be a help or a hindrance, or may do nothing at all for your weight-loss programme. In this chapter we take a brief look at drugs that may contribute to weight gain, then review some of the herbs and supplements that are often mentioned as helpful for weight loss and fat burning.

DRUGS THAT MAY PROMOTE WEIGHT GAIN

There are a number of drugs that can actually *cause* weight gain. It's important to read through the complete list of side-effects for all drugs prescribed for you. If weight gain is listed as a possible side-effect, discuss with your doctor whether there are any options that are more diet-friendly. (Don't, however, go off any prescribed medication. You should always discuss any changes to your medication with your practitioner.)

Some of the drugs that may contribute to weight gain include:

- steroid anti-inflammatories
- lithium
- oestrogen and progesterone independently, or together as in the contraceptive Pill

- antidiabetes drugs, like insulin
- various antidepressants, especially Prozac
- mood-stabilizing and anticonvulsant drugs such as those given for bipolar disorder, including lithium and carbamazepine
- beta blockers
- sedatives
- tranquillizers.

SUPPLEMENTS AND HERBS

There are literally hundreds of vitamins, herbs, minerals, enzymes, essential fatty acids and combination-formula supplements that promote themselves as being helpful in:

- increasing metabolism or making it more effective
- aiding fat-burning
- slowing fat storage
- balancing blood sugar
- reducing appetite.

Do they work? That's a good question, because many of the supplements have never been extensively studied. Some have undergone various studies and trials, and others have been in use for centuries as part of traditional Chinese medicine or Ayurvedic remedies. There are also some that are touted mainly on the basis of anecdotal evidence. And then there is the constant battery of hype, with never-ending infomercials, bus shelter adverts, magazine and newspaper adverts and multilevel marketers trying to sell you the latest 'miracle diet' supplement – the one that will finally melt the pounds off while you sleep, or allow you to eat anything and still lose weight, or rev up your metabolism and burn 50 per cent more fat!

I'll let you in on a big secret. That miracle diet supplement doesn't exist. I get a thousand e-mails a week from frustrated thyroid patients who are trying to lose weight, and I guarantee you, if any of these pills worked, I would be hearing from the legions of people who were thrilled with their miracle pills. So far, I haven't heard from any. And yes, here and there I've fallen prey to the marketing claims and tried a bottle or two of miracle pills myself. They haven't solved the problem. No matter what, I'm always back to diet and exercise.

That said, there are some supplements and herbs that *may* help you in your weight-loss efforts. I emphasize *may*, because there are no guarantees, and some supplements will do nothing at all for you; some might actually do the opposite (and you'll be one of the few people who gains weight on something that is supposed to help!). Some of the supplements, however, might actually be a great fit for you and help with your weight-loss efforts.

For each supplement, I've provided my recommendation regarding whether it might be worth trying. Keep in mind that many combination supplements for weight loss contain various ingredients, so you may see some products that contain a number of these supplements together in one pill or liquid formula.

5-HTP

5-hydroxytryptophan (5-HTP) is a precursor to the neurotransmitter serotonin. There is some evidence that 5-HTP may be able to reduce appetite and promote weight loss. One trial showed increased weight loss among overweight women who took 600 to 900 mg of 5-HTP daily. Another study found that people with Type II diabetes significantly reduced their carbohydrate and fat intake after several weeks of taking 750 mg per day of 5-HTP. Other studies have found that 5-HTP taken at a daily dose of 8 mg per kilogram body weight could reduce overall caloric intake without a person having to make any particular effort to cut food intake. It was thought that the 5-HTP increases a sense of fullness. In addition to weight loss, 5-HTP is also thought to help with late afternoon and evening cravings.

Recommendation: Worth trying, but check with your practitioner regarding any potential interactions with antidepressants or other drugs.

7-KETO

7-KETO (3-acetyl-7-oxo-dehydroepiandrosterone) is related to DHEA. One study found that, when taken alongside a somewhat calorie-restricted diet with exercise, 7-KETO resulted in greater weight loss and body fat reductions than a placebo. It's thought that 7-KETO may be able to help make T4 to T3 conversion more effective, resulting in higher T3 levels.

Recommendation: May be worth trying, but keep in mind that it's a hormone precursor, so tread carefully.

Acetyl-L-Carnitine

Acetyl-L-carnitine is thought to have the following functions:

- **helps the hypothalamus stimulate production of growth hormone during sleep**
- **helps to reduce leptin resistance**
- **speeds the burning of fat by delivering more fat into the mitochondria.**

Carnitine links with fat and moves it into the mitochondria – the cell's furnace, or power plant – for burning, converting fats and carbohydrates into energy. Low carnitine is thought to slow delivery and allow extra fat to accumulate. One study found that people on a diet and exercise programme who also took 1,000 mg of acetyl-L-carnitine daily for 3 months lost significantly more weight than those who took a placebo. Some experts recommend taking 3,000 to 5,000 mg just once daily, around an hour before exercise to help burn fat during a workout.

Recommendation: Consider adding this supplement to your programme.

Alpha-Lipoic Acid

Alpha-lipoic acid is a powerful antioxidant that plays a role in helping to trigger production of adenosine triphosphate (ATP) to produce cellular energy. There is also some evidence that it may help to reduce insulin resistance and control blood sugar.

Recommendation: Consider adding this supplement to your programme.

Caffeine

Caffeine, whether in the form of coffee, caffeine pills or added as an ingredient to diet pills, is a popular weight-loss aid. Unfortunately, caffeine has a variety of side-effects, including elevated blood pressure, heart palpitations (particularly in people who have mitral valve prolapse), nervousness, irritability, sleeplessness and occasionally rapid heartbeat. It also is not particularly effective on its own, but appears to have the ability to enhance the thermogenic effect of other supplements. Like all stimulants, too, you lose the effects when you cut back or stop the levels, and you'll regain weight.

You need to be particularly careful about overuse of caffeine, particularly supplements that contain caffeine in its various forms. Some weight-loss formulas, for example, contain more than 300 mg of caffeine per 2-pill dosage (the same amount of caffeine that's in 2 to 3 strong cups of coffee) and can contain other stimulants such as yerba maté, guarana, green tea, Tibetan ginseng, panax ginseng, cocoa nut and kola nut – most of which contain caffeine. While the recommended maximum daily intake is 450 mg of caffeine per day total, the recommended dosages of these weight-loss formulas suggest taking up to 6 capsules a day, which would provide almost 1,000 mg of caffeine – an amount that could trigger a variety of symptoms in many people.

Caffeine is a drug, and you can overdose on it. Symptoms of overdose range from insomnia to thirst, confusion, irregular heartbeat, dizziness and even convulsions and breathing problems. Particularly when you're taking supplements that contain caffeine, then adding caffeine from coffee, tea, foods and other medicines, you can easily get into a danger zone.

Recommendation: Except for a few cups of coffee or green tea, use at your own risk.

Calcium

Calcium appears to have a connection to weight loss, although studies tend to show that this connection is to calcium-rich dairy foods. However, it's still important to ensure that you get sufficient calcium, and 1,000 to 2,000 mg a day can be particularly helpful. Some experts recommend using calcium citrate-malate and calcium carbonate forms.

Recommendation: Add this supplement to your programme.

Capsaicin/Cayenne Pepper

A slight reduction in appetite has been seen with the consumption of approximately 10 grams of cayenne pepper along with meals. Similar amounts are also thought to have the ability to increase metabolism of dietary fats and suppress appetite. Capsaicin is the ingredient in cayenne pepper that is thought to have this effect, and it can be taken in supplement form.

Recommendation: Consider adding this food or supplement to your programme.

Chitosan

Chitosan is made from the shells of shellfish. The idea behind chitosan is that it binds to fat and prevents you from absorbing the fat, making it pass through your body. It's a popular ingredient in many of the so-called 'fat-blocker' supplements. There is not much in the way of evidence that chitosan actually works for fat absorption, but as a fibre supplement it appears to help with reducing cholesterol levels in some people.

Recommendation: Save your money.

Chromium Picolinate

The mineral chromium in the form called chromium picolinate has had interesting but inconsistent results. Some studies have shown that it has no effect on weight loss but can help maintain muscle during weight loss. There is growing evidence that chromium can help in improving blood sugar control in people with Type II diabetes or insulin resistance by improving the body's responsiveness to insulin. There have been some questions regarding whether chromium picolinate may cause DNA damage, however, but this is controversial and as yet undecided. The dosage range for insulin control is as high as 1,000 mcg daily.

Recommendation: Worth trying, but keep track of developments regarding any downsides.

Coenzyme Q-10

Coenzyme Q-10 (CoQ-10) is a soluble antioxidant that helps the cells' mitochondria – the powerhouse – to generate nearly all of the energy that the cells need to function. It's thought that sufficient levels of CoQ-10 are needed for optimum energy and functional metabolism. A 200-mg-a-day dose is considered the minimum.

Recommendation: Good antioxidant, can't hurt and might help.

Coleus

Although there are no specific clinical trials, there is clinical support for use of the herb coleus for weight loss. *Coleus forskolin* supplements in the 50- to 100-mg range can be taken two to three times per day, and the herb is also thought to have thyroid-supportive effects.

Recommendation: Might be worth trying.

Conjugated Linoleic Acid/CLA

One supplement thought to help not with weight loss but with reducing fat storage and increasing muscle mass is conjugated linoleic acid (CLA). Conjugated linoleic acid is the name for a group of fatty acids found in dairy products (except fat-free dairy products) and some meats. CLA has largely been removed from our diets over the last 50 years, due to changes in livestock development and feeding practices.

Studies published by the American Chemical Society, the *Journal of International Medical Research*, the *Journal of Nutrition*, the *International Journal of Obesity* and *Lipids* have found that taking CLA can help with reducing body fat while increasing lean muscle mass. There is evidence that CLA acts to indirectly spur the metabolism to store less fat, which prevents fat from being deposited into the body, thereby reducing body fat mass. It's also thought that CLA can help with leptin resistance and can reduce the inflammatory signals coming out of fat cells.

Studies have shown that 3 to 4 grams (3,000 to 4,000 mg) per day of CLA can help with muscle mass, and 6 grams a day can help with insulin levels. One double-blind, randomized, placebo-controlled study found that CLA reduces fat and preserves muscle tissue. An average reduction of 6 pounds of body fat was found in the group that took CLA compared to a placebo group. The study found that approximately 3.4 grams of CLA per day is needed to obtain the beneficial effects.

CLA has been the subject of a variety of research in the past several years, and findings also suggest that some of the other benefits of CLA include the following:

- increases metabolic rate – this would obviously be a positive benefit for thyroid patients, as hypothyroidism – even when treated – can reduce the metabolic rate in some people.
- decreases abdominal fat – adrenal imbalances and hormonal shifts that are common in thyroid patients frequently cause rapid accumulation of abdominal fat, so this benefit could be quite helpful.
- enhances muscle growth – muscle burns fat, which also contributes to increased metabolism, thus being useful in weight loss and management.
- lowers cholesterol and triglycerides – since many thyroid patients have elevated cholesterol and triglyceride levels, even with treatment, this benefit can have an impact on a thyroid patient's health.
- lowers insulin resistance – insulin resistance is a risk for some hypothyroid patients, and lowering it can also help prevent adult-onset diabetes and make it easier to control weight.

All CLA is not created equal, and it's not recommended that you get a cut-rate brand. You're better off using the patented form of CLA known as Tonalin, which is found in a number of brands. Tonalin is the formulation that has been scientifically tested.

Some people report feeling slightly queasy after taking CLA, or have stomach pain or even loose stools. To minimize side-effects, CLA should be taken with a protein; milk is often recommended. Side-effects usually go away after 2 weeks of taking the supplement.

When I first began taking CLA (4,000 mg a day), there were 2 or 3 days the first week when I felt slightly green, but I began to take it with a bit of milk, which eliminated the problem. After just 1 week, I noticed less abdominal bloating and a slight reduction in appetite, which may be a result of lower blood sugar. After 3 weeks, my abdominal fat pouch shrunk substantially. Other fat areas (such as cheeks, upper arms, bottom) seemed to be slowly reducing as well. I found that CLA worked very well for the first 2 months in terms of spot reducing some areas of fat, especially my abdomen and face. But after a few months, its effects seemed to slow down for me; some patients have reported a similar slowdown. Others have reported continued success with CLA.

A handful of people have reported to me that CLA had the opposite effect on them and was actually making them feel more bloated and possibly causing weight gain. If this happens to you, you should obviously discontinue it.

Recommendation: Definitely give this a try to see if it helps.

DHEA

There are some clinical trials showing that dehydroepiandrosterone (DHEA) supplementation can lower fat mass without reducing total body weight. DHEA supplementation should typically not be done without testing your DHEA levels beforehand, however, as too much DHEA can cause a variety of symptoms, especially in women, including facial hair and acne.

Recommendation: Can be a tremendous help, but only take if you're tested and shown to be DHEA deficient.

Ephedra/Ephedrine/Ma Huang

Ephedra sinica, commonly known as ma huang, is a central nervous system stimulant that was at one time a common ingredient in many weight-loss and diet supplements. You may still be able to find ephedra in some selected weight-loss formulations in some traditional Chinese medicine remedies. In the past, ephedra was frequently combined with caffeine – a combination that has sometimes been referred to as herbal Phen-Fen – for greater effectiveness.

There is no question that the ephedra/caffeine combination helps promote weight loss in the short term. Unfortunately, these supplements were shown to have particularly dangerous side-effects. In just a several-year period, the US Food & Drug Administration (FDA) reportedly had records showing at least 70 deaths and more than 14,000 adverse events linked to ephedra use, including strokes, heart attacks, seizures, psychiatric and psychotic episodes, nausea, vomiting, autonomic hyperactivity and heart palpitations.

Supporters argue that ephedra has been used safely for centuries, and it's true. Ma huang has been used in Chinese medicine for centuries, though not in combination with caffeine and not at the doses – or overusage – seen with the weight-loss supplements. Ultimately, most people who used ephedra products gained the weight back quickly, because the artificial increase in metabolism enjoyed while taking these drugs did not last.

Recommendation: You probably shouldn't use these products.

Garcinia Cambogia/Hydroxycitric Acid

Garcinia cambogia is a tree whose tropical fruit contains high amounts of the compound hydroxycitric acid (HCA). It's thought that HCA may be able to help inhibit the conversion of sugar into fat, curb appetite and reduce sweet cravings. There are also claims that HCA can reduce the amount of excess carbohydrates that get converted to body fat. Research shows, however, that the supplement has little effect. While HCA is a common ingredient in many weight-loss supplements, the evidence is primarily anecdotal, but the supplement is considered safe with no side-effects.

Recommendation: Probably ought to save your money.

Glucosol

Glucosol is derived from the crepe myrtle tree native to southern Asia. The main ingredient, corosolic acid, has been shown in a variety of studies to support natural glucose metabolism and to activate cell glucose-transporter mechanisms that balance blood glucose levels. Corosolic acid also continues to work for a time after the treatment is stopped. In one study, Glucosol at daily dosages of 48 mg for 2 weeks showed a significant reduction (as much as 30 per cent) in blood glucose levels.

Recommendation: Definitely worth trying, but talk to your doctor first if you're hypoglycaemic or have diabetes.

Glutamine/L-Glutamine

Glutamine is an amino acid that is usually abundant in the body and is stored in muscle. There is a theory that sometimes the body's need for glutamine is greater than its ability to make it, particularly when you are exercising and building muscle. Glutamine is thought to help protect muscles and reduce cravings for carbohydrates like sweets, starches and alcohol.

Recommendation: Consider trying this, especially if you're doing weight-bearing and muscle-building exercise.

Green Tea Extract

Both green tea and its extract are rich in polyphenols (epigallocatechin gallate, or EGCG), which may help your weight-loss programme by increasing energy expenditure and thermogenesis (the increase in body heat that results from digestion, absorption and metabolization of food). In one study, healthy young men who took two green tea capsules (containing 50 mg of caffeine and 90 mg of EGCG) three times a day had a significantly greater energy expenditure and fat oxidation than those who took caffeine alone or placebo. There are claims that drinking green tea in liquid form can also be a help in weight loss. Downsides of green tea extract are that it may make you jittery, give you headaches, or even cause insomnia.

Recommendation: Green tea may be a better way to get your caffeine fix, but don't overdo it, and be careful if you're caffeine sensitive.

Guarana

The herb guarana contains caffeine, along with theobromine and theo-phylline, which are all thought potentially to curb appetite and increase weight loss. Guarana has 30 per cent more caffeine than coffee, so you should be particularly careful about supplementing with it because it can be overstimulating, especially when combined with other sources of caffeine (e.g. gotu kola, or straight caffeine itself) in some weight-loss combination formula supplements.

Recommendation: Too much caffeine, and not a good idea for most.

Gymnema Sylvestre

Gymnema sylvestre is an Ayurvedic herbal remedy that is thought to help particularly with reducing sweet cravings and minimizing sugar absorption in the intestines.

Recommendation: Not enough research to really recommend it at this time.

Hoodia Gordonii

Hoodia gordonii is a supplement derived from a cactus found in the deserts of the Kalahari in southern Africa. Pharmaceutical researchers claim hoodia contains a substance known as P57 that acts like glucose with nerve cells in the brain and tricks the body into thinking it's full. Drug companies are reportedly developing drugs using hoodia that may be released in the future, but the pure form of the herb supposedly has appetite-suppressant capabilities. There aren't any side-effects or dangers to hoodia, and while the research is preliminary, it's promising. You need a pure hoodia supplement, not a weight-loss formula that contains a smaller amount of hoodia as an ingredient.

Recommendation: I've been using hoodia regularly and have found it a tremendous help in reducing appetite.

Milk Thistle

Milk thistle is a fat-burning herb that helps support the liver and detoxification. It is a common ingredient in detoxification and weight-loss formulas. Not much research has been done on this herb to establish the validity of claims, but anecdotally and clinically it is popular with many practitioners.

Recommendation: Considered fairly safe, but the jury is out on effectiveness.

Pantethine

Pantethine is a form of vitamin B_5 – pantothenic acid. It's been shown to help reduce triglyceride levels and to reduce abdominal and visceral fat and obesity. The optimum dose to help with metabolizing fat appears to be 600 to 900 mg daily.

Recommendation: Definitely worth trying.

Phaseolus Vulgaris/Starch Blockers

Beans can partially interfere with the body's ability to digest carbohydrates. (This is actually why they cause so much gas!) Based on this knowledge, a variety of products containing the French white bean *Phaseolus vulgaris* have been marketed as carbohydrate blockers. However, there is no specific evidence that supplements made from this treatment (or any other bean) actually aid in weight loss.

Recommendation: Save your money.

Pyruvate

Pyruvate is a compound in the body that is also found in particular fruits and vegetables. It's thought that pyruvate may increase resting metabolism slightly, can help with overall endurance and can slightly accelerate fat loss. One trial found that pyruvate at 22 to 44 grams per day could enhance weight loss and help reduce body fat for overweight adults eating a low-fat diet. Several trials using lower doses – from 6 to 10 grams per day – along with exercise, showed similar results with weight loss and body fat. Much of the research was done based on 20 to 30 grams per day, but it's thought that 5 grams per day is enough to produce results.

Recommendation: There's enough evidence to make this worth trying.

Spirulina

Spirulina, a type of algae, is a source of protein and a variety of other nutrients. In one double-blind trial, overweight people who took 2.8 grams of spirulina three times per day for 4 weeks experienced a very small and insignificant weight loss. Thus, although spirulina had been promoted as a weight-loss aid, the scientific evidence supporting its use for this purpose is weak.

Recommendation: The jury is still out.

Taurine

Taurine is one of the lesser-known amino acids and has a number of different functions in the body. It aids the liver in forming bile acids, helps with detoxification of toxins and toxic chemicals from the body, and is even thought to help reduce chemical sensitivity. It is also a good diuretic. Doses of 500 to 1,000 mg daily of taurine are considered safe and effective.

Recommendation: Worth trying.

Vitamin C

Vitamin C may be able to help with weight loss in those who are significantly overweight. The main risks of too much vitamin C – that is, more than 2,000 mg a day – are diarrhoea or loose bowels and abdominal cramping.

One research team found that resting metabolism before and after an infusion of vitamin C among people between 60 and 74 years old resulted in resting metabolism increases, on average, of almost 100 calories per day. So people burned 100 more calories on the days after vitamin C infusion without doing anything else different.

Some experts recommend that you take vitamin C 'to bowel tolerance'. Basically, you start with 500 mg a day and keep adding 500 mg a day until you get to a point where you have diarrhoea. Then cut back to the highest level that will not cause stomach problems. Take that daily dose, which for many can be as much as 5,000 mg (or 5 grams).

Recommendation: Always a good supplement.

Zinc

Supplementation with selenium and zinc may be tried with lower-calorie diets to prevent decline of the thyroid hormone T3. You shouldn't take more than 400 mcg of selenium a day. A daily dose of 15 mg of zinc is helpful.

Recommendation: Worth trying.

MESOTHERAPY

While not really in the category of supplements, I felt it important to mention mesotherapy, which involves injecting a patient-specific mixture of natural extracts and chemicals into the *mesoderm*, the middle layer of the skin where cellulite resides. The technique is used for weight loss and spot fat reduction, as well as for sports injuries, cellulite, hair loss, skin conditions, chronic pain, bone spurs, allergies, arthritis, chronic fatigue and chronic sinus problems. Dr Michel Pistor pioneered the technique in France in 1952, where there are roughly 15,000 practitioners. Mesotherapy is practised extensively in the UK, France, Belgium, Italy, Germany, Switzer-land and South America, and French studies show the treatment is effective for weight loss.

The idea behind mesotherapy is that different chemicals, herbs or drugs are injected to help deal with the particular problem. In the case of cellulite reduction, for example, the practitioner will prepare a mixture that includes vasodilators (which improve blood flow to the area), stimulants for lymph flow and lipolytic agents (which break down fat tissue). Injections are given 4 to 6 millimetres below the skin surface with a special mesotherapy pistol. The injections increase blood and lymph flow in the cellulite area, and the broken-down fat is carried away and excreted by the body. Cellulite-reduc-tion patients may receive between 20 and 300 shots per session over 10 to 15 weekly visits. The procedure takes only a few minutes each visit.

Mesotherapy injections can be given directly into areas that need spot reduction such as love-handles, 'bra bulge', 'saddlebags', saggy neck and so on. Fat-burning mesotherapy can be done in the abdominal area to help reduce abdominal fat. Mesotherapy is not a substitute for weight loss, but it does appear to be a non-surgical solution for spot fat reduction, and some patients have reported that it greatly helped with weight loss. Singer Roberta Flack, herself hypothyroid, has been battling a weight problem for years. She has been seeing New York's Dr Bissoon, the practitioner who brought the therapy to the United States, and has lost more than 40 pounds with her mesotherapy treatments so far, along with a diet and exercise programme.

CHAPTER 7

Stress, Mind and Body

Drag your thoughts away from your troubles by
the ears, by the heels, or any other way, so you
can manage it; it's the healthiest thing a body
can do.

— MARK TWAIN

Your mind, emotions, stress level and brain chemistry have a tremendous ability to affect your health, symptoms and ultimately your body's ability to lose weight. In scientific terms, it's called neuro-endocrinology – that is, the relationship between your neurological system, comprised of the brain and nerves, and your endocrine system, consisting of the hormones. In simple terms, it's the mind–body relationship, and it's an important part of your overall efforts to achieve a healthy, lasting weight loss.

There are a number of mind–body challenges and brain chemistry issues that you should be aware of, all of them capable of derailing your weight-loss efforts if not identified and treated.

MIND/BODY/BRAIN CHEMISTRY CHALLENGES
Brain Hormones

Melatonin, a hormone produced by the brain's pineal gland, helps regulate sleeping and waking. Melatonin levels typically rise in the evening, stay high during the night, then decline in the morning as you wake up. Melatonin typically declines with age and can become almost undetectable in some older people. Reduced light during winter months also causes melatonin levels to remain unnaturally high, which makes you feel sleepy and can cause depression, fatigue and reduced activity. Some experts believe that low-dose melatonin supplementation (1–2 mg per night) can be safe and effective at helping replace low levels of melatonin. But long-term use of this hormone is still being assessed.

A sense of hunger can be intricately tied to your brain chemistry. Your hypothalamus senses you need energy and issues the various neurotransmitters including neuropeptide Y (NPY) that deliver one key message: Eat carbohydrates. The surge of NPY is what you experience as a sensation of hunger. Once the brain senses you've eaten enough carbohydrates, it releases serotonin to tell the body that you've had enough. This serotonin gives you a sense of well-being.

There are some situations, including illness, stress and depression, where your body may be unable to produce or detect serotonin. These chemical imbalances can interfere with your ability to lose weight, and these sorts of dysfunctions in the feedback system appear to be more common in people who have thyroid disease. In these cases, antidepressants can sometimes help restore the proper production of and response to serotonin.

Chronic Stress

When you are under chronic stress, you flood your body with cortisol – a hormone that stimulates appetite. At the same time, the increased adrenaline increases fatty acid and blood sugar levels, stimulating the body to store those extra calories primarily as fat in the deep abdominal area – the worst place to gain weight, from a health standpoint. The abdominal fat makes you more insulin resistant and produces various inflammatory markers that increase your risk of diabetes, insulin resistance and heart disease.

Poor self-image contributes to chronic stress. One survey found that 56 per cent of women and 43 per cent of men disliked their overall appearance. Not only does this sort of negative self-image add to chronic stress but it can damage your social, professional and sexual life – and create a weight-loss block.

One way to tell if chronic stress is contributing to your weight is your waist measurement. If you're a man with a waist size greater than 40 inches, or a woman with a waist wider than 35 inches, you're most likely at risk.

Using Food as a Drug

Many of us use food to medicate our stress or problems. We eat to alleviate stress, to feel comforted, to relax, to relieve frustration and boredom, to procrastinate, and even when we're really happy. Are you using food emotionally as therapy? If you feel that most problems can be made better by your favourite food, or that special occasions deserve special foods or treats, or if food makes you feel less angry or stressed, then you are likely an emotional eater. Part of successful weight loss is to identify emotional triggers that may cause you to eat, and find tools – besides a fork or spoon! – that can help defuse these triggers.

In his excellent book titled *Dr Bob Arnot's Revolutionary Weight Control Program*, Arnot actually compares food to recreational drugs:

> What's the difference between a diner downing a 16-ounce fat-drenched steak with onion rings and taking a slug of heroin? Dosage. Both are hitting brain cells with opiates ... Refined carbohydrates ... are digested quickly and cause a large rise in blood sugar. While you'll notice the fastest impact on serotonin levels, this is a short-lived strategy and can cause rapid gains in weight. These foods are the dietary equivalent of 'crack', since you'd have to hammer yourself all day long with them to keep feeling good.

Unfortunately, many people do get high on food all day long. A chocolate croissant and coffee for breakfast – pretty much mainlining sugar and caffeine. Then a sandwich with crisps or chips and a sugary cola for lunch – more carbohydrates and caffeine. Then a double latte and a giant cookie as an afternoon snack. Home for dinner of a big bowl of pasta followed by a bowl of microwave popcorn in front of the television. It's an all-day carbohydrate/caffeine festival. Some even add nicotine to the mix for extra stimulation when the sugar highs wear off.

People who eat like this – and there are many out there! – are using food to help manipulate their brain chemistry and hormones. And, if it works well enough, it's possible to become addicted to the hit of 'drugs' from various types of foods and ways of eating. Obviously, eating this way is a major impediment to weight loss.

MIND/BODY/BRAIN CHEMISTRY SOLUTIONS
A New Attitude

First, you need to confront your inner critic and stop talking to yourself negatively. You would never put up with someone else telling you that you are fat, unattractive, lazy, worthless, or any of the other negatives you may be heaping on yourself due to your weight.

Secondly, find a part of your body that you *do* like, and regularly praise yourself. It doesn't matter whether it's your terrific-looking feet, really great eyes or best-shaped calves in town – just pick one part of your body and continually tell yourself how terrific that part is. If you like even one part of yourself, it's a start.

Thirdly, stop putting your life on hold simply because you want to lose weight. Many of us make weight loss into some sort of oasis in the desert that we are travelling towards.

When I lose weight, I'll start going swimming again.
When I lose weight, I'll reunite with my old friend.
When I lose weight, I'll make an effort to find a new romance.
When I lose weight, we'll finally schedule the wedding.
When I lose weight, I'll finally try to get a new job.
And so on …

Life is too short to keep putting everyone and everything on hold until some day in the future when you achieve your 'perfect' weight. Give yourself permission to live, make changes and do the things you enjoy *today!*

Herbal Solutions

There are a variety of herbs that can aid in mind–body balancing. Reducing stress should be one of your most important mind–body goals in terms of your overall weight-loss programme. Holistic physician Hyla Cass, co-author of *Natural Highs*, shares these herbal and supplement suggestions for relaxation:

> You can start with kava 60–75 mg (kavalactones), increasing to two if that's what works for you. If you still don't feel relaxed, try, or add, any of the following, preferably one at a time to gauge your response. (If you do end up taking them all, reduce the dose of each by one-half, or take a combination formula.)

- Take about 60 mg of valerian
- 100 mg of hops
- 100 mg of passionflower
- 500 mg of GABA
- 500 mg of taurine

One herbal formula developed by holistic physician Jacob Teitelbaum combines many of the above components. Teitelbaum's specially formulated Fatigued to Fantastic!® Revitalizing Sleep Formula functions as a herbal sleep aid. It can also work as a daytime supplement for relaxation and stress reduction. It contains valerian, passionflower, L-theanine, hops, wild lettuce and Jamaica dogwood, which help with relaxation and healthful sleep if taken at night-time. I have found this formulation particularly helpful during times when I'm under more stress than usual, or nights when I'm finding it difficult to get to sleep.

For balancing brain chemistry, you may want to consider supplements known as CraniYums, which claim to help people stay on their diets by safely and effectively increasing the brain's natural appetite, mood and energy regulators (the neurotransmitters serotonin and dopamine). I've tried them and they do seem to help with cravings, especially carbohydrate cravings.

When it comes to depression, remember that serious clinical depression or bipolar disease needs to be overseen and treated by a doctor. If you are experiencing significant symptoms of depression or anxiety, see your practitioner for guidance.

If you are in a down mood, there are some herbal supplements that can help pick you up, energize you and help lift minor depression. Cass suggests these herbal and supplemental natural mood lifters:

- 100 mg of pantothenic acid (B_5)
- 20 mg of pyridoxine (B_6)
- 10 mcg of B_{12}
- 100 mcg of folic acid
- 50 mg of 5-HTP (increasing gradually to 300 mg)
- 300–900 mg of St John's Wort (According to Dr Cass, it may take a few days or even weeks for St John's Wort to kick in, but it's worth the wait.)

Dr Cass also suggests that the following products can be added one at a time to see how you respond:

- 500 mg of tyrosine
- 500 mg of DL Phenylalanine (DLPA)
- 200 mg of S-adenosylmethionine (SAMe)
- 600 mg of trimethyl glycine (TMG)
- 40 mg of niacin (B_3)

Prescription Drugs

When it comes to dealing with depression or anxiety, there are a number of prescription drugs that can be used. Depression that doesn't respond to herbal or natural remedies may warrant use of an antidepressant medication. If you're dealing with excess weight and are considering taking an antidepressant, be sure to discuss with your prescribing practitioner that you want one of the medications that isn't likely to cause more weight gain.

While every patient is different and there are reports of people gaining and/or losing weight on every single different antidepressant, the drugs considered least likely to generate weight gain include nefazodone (Dutonin) and venlafaxine (Efexor). The Prozac-type medications may cause some short-term weight loss, but in the long term they tend to cause weight gain in some people.

Stress-Reduction Drugs

Sometimes anxiety is chronically debilitating. At this point, some doctors would recommend medication. The medications used most often to treat anxiety include:

- certain selective serotonin reuptake inhibitors (SSRIs) such as paroxetine hydrochloride (Seroxat)
- tricyclic antidepressants such as imipramine hydrochloride (Tofranil) and clomipramine hydrochloride (Anafranil)
- benzodiazepines such as alprazolam (Xanax), diazepam (Valium), lorazepam (Ativan) and clonazepam (Rivotril).

Some of these medications can be addictive and have a variety of side-effects, so be sure to discuss with your practitioner any plans to take an anti-anxiety drug. Talk about your options and the pros and cons of various drugs before you decide.

Cognitive Behaviour Techniques

Cognitive behaviour therapy is not about sitting on a therapist's couch for years exploring early childhood experiences. It is practical and solution orientated, with the goal of helping you to rework the way you think about and therefore react to different situations. It is particularly helpful for people who are attempting to lose weight or maintain weight loss. There are a number of specific behavioural strategies you can learn and practise with the aid of a therapist or support group:

- Tracking – self-monitoring of your eating habits and physical activity in an objective way through observation and recording is an important part of behaviour therapy. You can keep track of the amount and types of food you eat, calories and nutrient composition as well as the frequency, intensity and type of physical activities. For even more insight, keep track of your feelings and motivations to eat and exercise. Reviewing these records will help you gain insight into your own eating and exercise patterns and habits. You may also be able to identify particular situations such as boredom or frustration that trigger your worst episodes of unhealthy eating.

- **Stimulus control** – identifying situations that may encourage you to eat poorly enables you to limit your exposure to high-risk situations. Examples of stimulus-control strategies include learning to shop carefully for healthy foods, keeping high-calorie foods out of the house, limiting the times and places of eating and consciously avoiding situations where you are likely to overeat.

- **Problem solving** – involves looking at problem areas you have in terms of eating and physical activity, brainstorming possible solutions and evaluating outcomes of possible changes in behaviour. For example, some people who are veteran snackers while watching television have taken up new habits, such as keeping needlework, crossword puzzles or manicure supplies to hand to replace snacking.

- **Rewards** – you can help change your own behaviour by using rewards for specific actions, such as rewarding yourself for increasing time spent exercising, or rewarding yourself for cutting consumption of particular foods. Self-rewards can be monetary (e.g. putting aside money for a special item or buying yourself something you've wanted) or social (e.g. going to the cinema).

- **Cognitive restructuring** – you may have unrealistic goals or inaccurate beliefs about weight loss and body image, such as 'I can lose 10 pounds in 2 weeks!' 'I'm not attractive unless I'm a size 8.' 'Women don't think men are sexy unless they have a six-pack.' If so, you need to change self-defeating thoughts and feelings that undermine weight-loss efforts. Cognitive therapy helps you come up with rational responses to replace negative thoughts. For example, 'I blew my diet this morning by eating that doughnut; I may as well eat what I like for the rest of the day' could be replaced by 'Well, I ate the doughnut this morning, but I can still eat in a healthy manner at lunch and dinner.'

Getting 'Inhibited'

According to research published in the *American Journal of Clinical Nutrition*, what's known as your inhibition when it comes to eating snacks and high-calorie foods is linked to your likelihood of being overweight. In the Tufts University study, three specific behaviours – restraint, disinhibition and hunger – were examined in a group of more than 600 women.

Restraint is being able to reduce and restrict your food intake in order to maintain or lose weight.

Disinhibition is a tendency to eat too much when something tempting is there or when there are other factors that reduce your inhibitions (e.g. stress or fatigue), whether or not you are hungry.

Hunger is simply your sensitivity to feelings that you need food.

Interestingly, the researchers found that the higher the level of disinhibition, the higher the weight. Disinhibition eating is very strongly linked to obesity. The researchers told Reuters Health that being disinhibited about food also typically added up to weight gain of 30 pounds or more over 25 years, up to about age 60.

People who are disinhibited constantly face the desire to eat everything offered to them, or to eat an entire serving or large portion of a desirable food. Instead, however, it's best to practise restraint. Stop and ask yourself very specifically: 'Am I hungry?' If you decide you truly *are* hungry, have a small portion or taste, then stop. Being a restrained eater can help to minimize the negative effects of disinhibition.

When I read about this study, it was as if the researchers were speaking to me! My father's side of the family is Armenian/Assyrian – a culture where food is love, celebration, hospitality, comfort and medicine. I can't even imagine walking into my father's house without food being offered. After breakfast, the discussion is what you're going to eat for lunch. And before lunch is cleared away, we're talking about dinner. When I'm with my family, I start thinking 'Why not eat? I deserve to celebrate, relax and enjoy myself.' I go into full disinhibition mode.

I imagine many of you come from similar families, where food is used to express so many things and the idea of pushing away from the table when there's something good to eat is unheard of. It's tempting to think this is your background and you're doomed to live just like your family. But it's not so. Interestingly, I'm married to Mr Restrained Eater. He and his family eat when they are hungry, and then only what's needed. Certainly they celebrate a special occasion at a restaurant and make birthday cakes – they are not austere. But most of the time, they eat to live rather than live to eat.

Even if you grew up and are right now a full-scale disinhibited eater, after a few weeks of restrained eating, it becomes second nature. The cravings fade, especially for sweets and starchy carbohydrates like bread and rice, and you get in the groove of eating to live. I rarely have to stop and think about whether I'm hungry, because my blood sugar is balanced. I know exactly what I'm going to eat most days, how much and how many portions I can eat and whether I need to get in more vegetables, fruit, protein and so on, before the day is through, in order to complete my day's totals.

Even if you're currently in disinhibition mode, stop the next time you automatically reach for something high-calorie or high-fat, or are presented with a large portion of food, and ask yourself if you're actually hungry. It's a simple but very powerful technique to get started towards healthier eating.

Sleep

Sleep is absolutely essential to weight loss. Studies suggest that sleep loss may increase hunger and affect the body's metabolism, which may make it more difficult to maintain or lose weight. Specifically, the less sleep you get, the more cortisol is released. And cortisol stimulates hunger. At the same time, insufficient sleep may interfere with the body's ability to metabolize carbohydrates and may cause high blood levels of glucose, leading to higher insulin levels and greater fat storage. Inadequate sleep also drives down leptin levels, and low levels of leptin cause the body to crave carbohydrates.

One important study published in the journal *Lancet* in 1999 showed that, even in young, healthy people, a sleep deficit of 3 to 4 hours a night over the course of a week had a triple-whammy effect on the body, interfering with the ability to process carbohydrates, manage stress and maintain a proper balance of hormones. In the study, the men (aged 18 to 27) spent 16 consecutive nights in a clinical research centre. For the first 3 nights they spent 8 hours in bed; for the next 6 nights they stayed in bed for 4 hours; for the last 7 nights they were in bed for 12 hours. During the sleep-restricted second week, the men showed a substantial loss in their ability to process glucose, accompanied by a rise in insulin. In fact, insulin rose so much that the men had levels associated with a prediabetes state.

Dr Michael Thorpy, director of the Sleep-Wake Disorders Center at Montefiore Medical Center in New York, has said,

> Sleep loss is associated with striking alterations in hormone
> levels that regulate the appetite and may be a contributing
> factor to obesity. Any[one] ... making a resolution to lose
> weight ... should probably consider a parallel commitment for
> getting more sleep.

In addition to changes in sleep quantity, reductions in sleep *quality* can also affect weight. For example, decreased amounts of restorative deep or slow-wave sleep have been associated with significantly reduced levels of growth hormone – a protein that helps regulate the body's proportions of fat and muscle.

Dr John Winkelman, medical director of the Sleep Health Center at Brigham and Women's Hospital, and assistant professor of psychiatry at Harvard Medical School, says,

> Sleep loss disrupts a complex and interwoven series of
> metabolic and hormonal processes and may be a contributing
> factor to obesity. What most people do not realize is that
> better sleep habits may be instrumental to the success of any
> weight management plan.

Unfortunately, many of us aren't getting the sleep we need. Researchers have found that fewer than one in three adults is getting 8 or more hours of sleep per night on weeknights. Many studies have shown that the majority of us need around 8 hours per night, or we start to suffer the effects of chronic sleep deprivation.

Getting sufficient sleep is essential. In addition to talking to your practitioner about the use of herbal and prescription sleep aids, here are some other tips on getting a good night's sleep:

- Regular exercise can help, but try to avoid exercise within 3 hours of bedtime because it can jazz you up too much.
- Avoid caffeine, nicotine and alcohol in the late afternoon and evening.
- If you have trouble sleeping at night, don't nap during the day.
- Establish a relaxing pre-sleep ritual such as a warm bath or a few minutes of reading.

- **Create a pleasant sleep environment. Make it as dark and quiet as possible.**
- **If you can't sleep, don't stay in bed. After 30 minutes, go to another room and do something else that is relaxing until you feel sleepy.**

Breathing

It goes by a variety of names. In yoga, it's *pranayama*, the art and science of breathing. In marketing language, it's Breathercise or Oxycise. Some fitness centres are even incorporating it into their programmes. Whatever you call it, a programme of deep breathing exercises that are designed to take in more oxygen and release more carbon dioxide with each breath seem to help people with hypothyroidism to lose weight.

We know that hypothyroidism affects the strength of the respiratory muscles. Hypothyroidism is also known to increase reactivity of the bronchial passages, even if you don't have asthma. Even when treated, a substantial percentage of people with hypothyroidism report shortness of breath, feeling like they're not getting enough oxygen, or even needing to yawn to get more air as continuing symptoms.

For many of us, the ability to take in and process oxygen may be forever changed once hypothyroidism sets in. Even when fully treated, I suspect that most of us still don't take in and process oxygen fully. That is why specific attention to breathing seems to help some people with hypothyroidism. And learning how to breathe is about as inexpensive as it can be. All you need is some air and a pair of lungs to start. And no one can say that learning to breathe better isn't good for you, thyroid problem or not.

Breathing experts point to numerous health benefits of systematic breathing practice, including increased oxygen delivery to the cells, which helps provide sufficient energy to fuel metabolism, improve digestion, decrease fatigue, create more energy, reduce stress and promote relaxation. If you're interested in trying out better breathing for yourself, you can start by learning deep abdominal breathing. Here's a simple breathing exercise to try:

- **Lay on your back, body relaxed. Put your hand on your abdomen. Take a deep, slow breath through your nose, filling your belly so that your hand rises.**

- Exhale slowly, letting all the air out of your belly.
- Inhale again, filling the abdomen until your hand rises.
- Again, exhale. Feel the breath energy rising from the abdomen to the throat and back down again to the abdomen.

You can start practising this deep abdominal breathing anywhere: sitting in the car, standing in a queue, taking a shower. It's a first step towards incorporating deep breathing into your daily life. Several times a day, stop and just focus on your breathing. Take a few deep abdominal breaths. Every time you feel tired, try taking five deep abdominal breaths. See if these ventures in breathing practice help you to feel a bit more energetic or alert. If you want to delve into breathing to help your metabolism, I strongly recommend breathing coach Pam Grout's *Jumpstart Your Metabolism*, a wonderful book that has everything you need to know.

More and more interest is now focusing on specialized yoga breathing techniques that have the ability to change the autonomic nervous system in various ways. For example, one study looked at three different pranayamas (yoga breathing techniques). One group did breathing in and out of the right nostril (the other nostril is pressed closed with a finger), one group did breathing in and out of the left nostril, and a third group did alternate nostril breathing. Yoga experts believe that these types of breathing help to balance the metabolism, generate increased energy, concentration and mood, and help to balance endocrine disorders. In one study, these practices were carried out as 27 respiratory cycles repeated 4 times a day over the course of a month. At the end of the month-long practice, the right-nostril pranayama group showed a 37 per cent increase in their baseline oxygen consumption. The left-nostril group showed a 24 per cent increase, and the alternate-nostril group showed an 18 per cent increase. The increase in oxygen consumption can help make the metabolism more efficient.

Here are brief guidelines on how to do nostril breathing:

- Sit on the floor in lotus position with your legs comfortably crossed, or on a couch or chair, making sure your spine and head are straight.
- Rest your right hand on your right knee or in your lap
- Place your index and middle fingers of your left hand at the centre of your eyebrows.
- Keep your right nostril open and close your left nostril with your thumb.

- Inhale slowly and deeply through your right nostril to the count of 4.
- Hold your breath for the count of 2.
- Exhale to the count of 4.

That is one cycle of nostril breathing. Repeat the cycle daily, starting with a 1- to 2-minute session and working up to several sessions of 10 minutes each.

Emotional Freedom Technique

In his best-selling book, *The No-Grain Diet*, Dr Joseph Mercola talks about a unique way to beat cravings: the emotional freedom technique (EFT). EFT is basically a form of body work that he has referred to as 'psychological acupressure', which can help battle a desire or craving for particular foods. It involves tapping on particular spots of the head and chest combined with affirmations.

EFT was created over a decade ago. It's based on the same general concepts that acupuncture and acupressure have relied on for 5,000 years – the idea that energy that flows through the body and regulates health can be channelled and directed to places where it is most needed physically and emotionally.

Tapping with the fingertips is used to input energy onto specific meridians on the head and chest while you think about your specific problem – whether it is a traumatic event, an addiction, a craving, a pain, or whatever – and voice positive affirmations. This combination of tapping the energy meridians and voicing positive affirmations is meant to clear the short-circuit – the emotional block – from your body's bioenergy system, thus restoring your mind and body's balance.

I had an opportunity to review Dr Mercola's free online EFT course, as well as the multi-DVD/video course he has produced on EFT and sells on his website and at seminars. After watching for about an hour, I found it pretty silly. But I had watched him walk through the technique several times on the DVD and try it on various volunteers who were taped at one of his in-person seminars, so I decided that I would try the EFT technique myself.

After watching for about an hour, I had mastered the tapping spots for EFT and figured out an affirmation that fit with a persistent eye tic problem. I followed the process, which took less than a minute. I stopped. I waited for the tic to start back up. No tic. I waited for a few minutes, fully expecting the tic to reoccur. No tic. I went back to watching the DVD, fully expecting that once I diverted my attention from the tic, it would come right back. I watched for another hour and no tic. Three months later, it still hasn't come back. A few weeks later when some heart palpitations were bothering me (I have mitral valve prolapse), I again thought about the EFT technique. I'd taken a beta blocker and done some relaxation exercise and nothing was helping. I tried EFT and, within minutes, my palpitations were gone. I've now also used EFT to deal successfully with a craving for chocolate, and to combat stress. I've used it on my husband and child for assorted ailments and stressors. It has worked every time.

Dr Mercola considers EFT one of the key principles of healthy diet and weight loss. According to Mercola, EFT may be helpful in a number of aspects of weight loss, including:

- getting rid of cravings for unhealthy foods
- motivating you to exercise or to overcome exercise obstacles
- enhancing energy
- minimizing joint and muscle pain
- stimulating metabolism
- changing the way you view your own body.

You can learn how to do EFT by reading the free manual at Dr Mercola's website (see Appendix A); you don't need to watch the DVDs or videos, as I did. But if you want to really delve into it more fully, they can take you to the next level.

Other Stress Reducers

There are a number of other ways to help relieve anxiety and stress, boost mood and balance brain chemistry to create the optimal mind–body connection for weight loss:

- Meditation – one effective healing/mind–body technique is meditation. According to the Center for Integrative Medicine at Thomas Jefferson University Hospital in Philadelphia, meditation training can help patients with chronic illnesses reduce symptoms and improve quality of life. Meditation training also helps patients cope with stress, have an improved sense of well-being, reduce body tension and increase clearness of thinking, which all benefit the immune system. Meditation has helped to lower blood pressure, clear up skin problems and increase melatonin levels. By using magnetic resonance imaging (MRI), researchers have established that meditation actually activates certain structures in the brain that control the autonomic nervous system.

- Light therapy – you need to make sure that you get sufficient exposure to light, especially during the darker winter months. During wintertime, get outside for at least an hour each day in the afternoon without wearing sunglasses. If you can't get that sort of natural light exposure, consider investing in a light box. Artificial lights have been used as a treatment for winter depression and seasonal affective disorder for more than a decade. Recently, powerful and portable 10,000 lux desktop light boxes have made light therapy even more convenient, and you need only 30 minutes a day, usually earlier in the day. These lights can help alleviate depression, increase energy and stimulate serotonin availability in the nervous system. I have a wonderful 10,000 lux lamp that sits right on my desk next to my computer. I turn it on for 30 minutes when I first go to my desk in the morning, and it has a remarkable effect on my energy and helps curb those winter carbohydrate cravings.

- Exercise – in addition to being good for metabolism and weight loss, exercise is a great stress reliever and mood enhancer – another reason to get on the running shoes and get outside for a midday walk (that way you get your daylight exposure and kill two birds …).

- Guided imagery – according to a leading guided imagery expert, therapist Belleruth Naparstek, your brain doesn't know the difference between something you actually see and something you imagine. So your body responds as strongly to an image as to the real thing. I am a devoted fan of Naparstek's excellent series of guided imagery health programmes. One of my favourites is her programme for weight loss, which you can get on audiotape or CD (see Appendix A). I frequently listen to it when I'm on the treadmill and it is very relaxing and inspiring. It motivates me to keep going! Naparstek has told *Prevention* magazine that guided imagery helps you 'get in under your mind's radar' so that you can persuade your body to do something. 'It may be to increase brain chemicals that make you feel calm and centered, decrease hormones that make you hungry, change the levels of biochemical components in your bloodstream that affect blood sugar, even build more immune system cells to fight everything from cancer to the common cold.'

CHAPTER 8

Exercise

In this age, which believes that there is a short cut to everything, the greatest lesson to be learned is that the most difficult way is, in the long run, the easiest.

– HENRY MILLER

When you are trying to lose weight, particularly with an underlying metabolic issue like thyroid disease, exercise has to be an essential part of your overall approach. I know that some of you are going to groan and swear to me that you have a friend, co-worker or relative who lost weight just dieting. And I believe it. Ultimately, for most people, it's easier to cut calories than add physical activity.

But the question is: Was that person also battling a thyroid problem? It may not seem fair, but you can't just cut out some calories and watch the pounds melt off. You'll have to work harder, and may still have less success than someone else eating and working out at a similar level. But if you include exercise in your programme, you will see results.

Calorie restriction alone does allow for some weight loss, but it slows, then stops and often rebounds back up again, as your metabolism slows down in response to the calorie reduction. To keep your metabolism efficient, or to make it even more efficient, you absolutely need exercise for many reasons.

First, when done properly and for a sufficient time, exercise can burn fat. During the first 15 to 20 minutes that you are exercising, glycogen (that's the sugar in your muscles) is burned for energy. As you continue exercising, the body turns to glucose and free fatty acids from the bloodstream for energy. At about the 30- to 40-minute point, the body starts burning fatty acids from stored fat. Studies have repeatedly shown that when you combine a moderate cutback in calories with regular physical activity, you're not only going to be more successful in achieving your weight goals but you're far more likely to keep the weight off.

Second, exercise is good for your heart and cholesterol levels. Getting your heart pumping makes it stronger and healthier. It helps reduce your risk of cardiovascular disease and stroke. It improves cholesterol levels and ratios, helps you live longer ... enough said.

Third, exercise reduces insulin levels. According to Jean-Pierre Despres, professor of medicine and physical education and director of the Lipid Research Center at Laval University Hospital in Quebec,

> Exercise is probably the best medication on the market to treat insulin resistance syndrome ... Our studies show that low-intensity, prolonged exercise – such as a daily brisk walk of 45 minutes to an hour – will substantially reduce insulin levels.

Fourth, weight-bearing exercises improve your muscle mass, which raises metabolism. The more muscle you have, the more calories you burn.

Fifth, aerobic exercise has a shorter but powerful effect on metabolism, giving you a burst of metabolic efficiency during the period after your exercise session.

Sixth, stretching exercises help improve your flexibility, reduce muscle/joint pain and improve your balance.

Seventh, according to Byron Richards, author of *Mastering Leptin*, exercise helps combat leptin and insulin resistance. Exercise can lower both leptin and markers for inflammation.

HOW MUCH DO YOU NEED TO DO TO LOSE WEIGHT?

One survey looked at the characteristics of those who were able to lose at least 30 pounds and keep it off for a year. On average, they ate a diet that was no more than approximately 24 per cent fat, and they expended an average of 2,827 calories a week on exercise. Most of us would need to walk about 28 miles a week to expend this amount of energy! (I'm not walking 28 miles a week, but I guess I should!)

Experts have recently said that healthy people with a body mass index of less than 25 – meaning that they are of normal weight – need 60 minutes of physical activity a day to maintain that weight and avoid excess gain. That is in addition to reducing calories and minimizing saturated fat and sugar in the diet.

Maybe I should repeat that. They're saying that 60 minutes a day is for someone who *hasn't* got a weight problem. So if you are overweight, you need to consider this as your starting point. Don't get me wrong. I'm not doing 60 minutes a day. I'm not even close. But it's my ultimate goal. And it needs to be yours, too … for life.

This does not mean you have to go to the gym for an hour and work out. It does not mean you have to jog through your neighbourhood for an hour. It means you need an hour of physical activity a day. That includes cardiovascular exercise, which can be a full aerobics class, 10 minutes of skip roping, or just 5 minutes of going up and down the stairs. It includes strength training, which could be a circuit on your gym's resistance machines, a 20-minute upper body workout, or even 10 push-ups during a TV advert. Exercise includes stretching. You can do a full Pilates class, or 10 minutes of yoga, or just a quick stretch at your desk. It also includes other physical activities such as the walking you do to get around, cleaning your house, washing your car, gardening and playing with your children.

I can almost guarantee that if you are overweight and have a thyroid problem, you are not getting an hour of physical activity a day. Even those of us who are active delude ourselves about how much exercise we're actually getting. Researchers doing a survey said that about two-thirds of those who were trying to lose weight claimed that they were increasing their physical activity. But only 21 per cent were exercising at least 150 minutes a week, which is the absolute minimum recommended for weight loss by some experts.

Overall, about a quarter of us do no form of leisure-time physical activity and half do fewer than 30 minutes of moderate activity a day. Only one in four is actually active for 30 minutes or more. It's no coincidence that most of those active people are not battling weight problems.

THYROID PATIENT CHALLENGES TO EXERCISING

Even most people who don't have thyroid disease aren't getting the amount of exercise they need. But thyroid patients face a number of additional challenges that can make it harder to exercise.

Muscle/Joint Pain

Pain in the muscles and joints is a common thyroid symptom and can persist even after treatment is optimized. There are several things you can do to help with this sort of pain so that you can exercise more effectively.

You can take a high-quality fish oil supplement (2 to 3 grams a day). I particularly like Enzymatic Therapy's Eskimo Oil because it has no fish 'burp' – that is, that terrible fishy aftertaste you get with some fish oil supplements.

Nonsteroidal anti-inflammatory drugs (NSAIDs), including over-the-counter options such as aspirin, ibuprofen (Motrin, Brufen) and naproxen sodium (Naprosyn) can be helpful with muscle and joint pain and autoimmune-related inflammation.

Fatigue

Being tired is one of the most common complaints of many thyroid patients. You may find that even after treatment you feel too tired to keep up with your daily activities, much less exercise. Once your thyroid treatment is optimized, there are several things you can do to help increase energy.

Get enough sleep. It seems an obvious solution, but most people aren't getting enough sleep. Only 30 per cent of adults are getting 8 or more hours of sleep per night on weeknights. I personally have to get 8 hours or my immune system slowly starts to degrade.

Another thing that can affect energy is a low dehydroepiandrosterone (DHEA) level. Before supplementing with DHEA, you should have your level assessed by your doctor. If it is low, supplementation (usually no more than 1–5 mg a day for women, and up to 25 mg a day for men, every other day, taken in the morning) can help greatly. In my case, at one point I experienced extreme fatigue in the afternoon; my doctor found that I had particularly low DHEA levels. Within a week after she put me on a regimen of 5 mg of DHEA, I had enough energy to exercise again.

If you are suffering from flagging energy, you need to make sure that you are getting enough B vitamins. Vitamin B_{12} is essential for energy. Consider taking a B complex plus B_{12} separately in a sublingual form (dissolves under the tongue) for maximum absorption.

Also consider using one of the adaptogenic herbs that can help with energy. These include:

- **royal maca**
- **Asian ginseng and Siberian ginseng**
- **rhodiola**
- **schizandra – a Chinese herb that is used for fatigue.**

Resist the temptation of a giant-size latte, multiple cups of coffee, or taking herbal energy supplements that have stimulants such as caffeine, ephedra, ma huang, guarana or gotu kola. These are all like stepping on the accelerator of your adrenal system while keeping the brakes on. You rev things up but don't go anywhere.

Body work and energy work, such as yoga, tai chi, qigong (pronounced chee-gung) and Reiki, can all help in adding and balancing energy. In qigong, tai chi and yoga, gentle movements are used to move energy along the energy pathways of the body. In Reiki, a practitioner helps open up energy channels. (Personally, I've found yoga and Reiki to be most beneficial to my energy.)

Hyla Cass, holistic physician and best-selling co-author of *Natural Highs*, offers these suggestions for natural energy boosters:

> You can start with Siberian ginseng (400 mg), licorice (500 mg), pantothenic acid (100 mg). (The last two are more for adrenal support than actual energy.) Or take the amino acid tyrosine or DLPA (500 mg). Depending on your response, you can add in any or all of the following to create your own personal energy formula, preferably one at a time to gauge your response. This can differ from day to day, too, depending on how you are feeling. If you do end up taking them all, reduce the dose of each accordingly, by about one-third to one-half:

- Take about 100 mg of Asian or American ginseng
- 300 mg of ashwaganda
- 3,000 mg of reishi mushroom
- 100 mg of rhodiola
- 100–250 mg of DLPA
- 100–250 mg of tyrosine.

You Think You're Too Overweight or Out of Shape

If you feel you are very overweight, you may not think that you can do much of anything in the way of exercise. It may seem daunting. Your body may feel stiff and inflexible and you don't want to end up in pain after just one exercise session. Exercise expert and About.com exercise guide Paige Waehner has these suggestions for how to get started:

> First, choose something accessible. Walking is usually a popular choice because you can do it anywhere, there's no learning curve and you don't need fancy equipment or gym memberships. Allow your body time to get used to what you're doing, and make regular activity a part of each day, whether it's just walking more than usual or taking the stairs when you normally don't. The more active you are, the more comfortable you'll be and the more energy you'll have to go further and longer.

Even if all you can do to get started is walk around the block once, do a few sit-ups, or lift a 2-pound hand weight a few times, that's enough. Slowly add more distance, more repetitions, or more weight. Don't try to run a mile or bench-press 100 pounds your first time out or you'll end up sore, miserable and swearing that you'll never exercise again! Waehner says,

> One of biggest problems I see with new exercisers is that they start out too hard. Most people want to start where they want to be rather than where they are, and that almost always leads to quitting. The best way to avoid that is to do what you're comfortable with and add on to that each week.

Lack of Motivation

Psychologist and motivational fitness coach David Junno has found that when thinking about starting an exercise programme, many people think primarily about how much work and discomfort are involved. This makes it easy to come up with excuses not to start or continue.

> There are two secrets to overcoming our resistance to doing exercise. The first is to focus on the benefits and the second is to gather evidence that refutes our negative perceptions. Not only should you remind yourself of the benefits of exercise, such as getting in shape, losing weight, better sleep, better health, looking better and improved sex life, but you need to find evidence of those benefits.

According to Junno, to convince yourself of the benefits of exercise, you have to do it for a period of time. But getting to that point is often the biggest challenge – and you'll need to exercise even when you don't feel like it. To help begin exercising despite not feeling like it, Junno shares this simple experiment:

> Establish an exercise routine, for example, taking a brisk 30-minute walk four times a week. Before you take each walk, rate how you feel about taking that walk. You can do this by using a 1 to 10 scale with 1 being the worst and 10 being the best. Then take your walk and afterwards rate the actual experience on your 1 to 10 scale. What do you notice? There is a good chance that you are going to rate the experience higher after you do it. Learning that doing exercise is going to feel a whole lot better than we anticipate, is a powerful way to combat the negative thinking that often gets in the way of our intentions.

Staying Motivated

Staying motivated can be a challenge to even the most regular exercises. Fitness expert and trainer Silvia Treves suggests that a few sessions with a personal trainer in the beginning can help. She explains,

> That way, you can learn the exact way to perform the exercises and movements and learn how to protect your spine, neck and back from injury. Clients tell me that they are likelier to continue working out if they don't always feel incredibly sore for days after exercising.

Some experts suggest following the 10-minute rule. When you don't feel like exercising, set your wristwatch alarm or a timer for 10 minutes at the start of your exercise session. If you want to quit after 10 minutes, then stop. But it's likely that, once you start, you'll be feeling pretty good and will continue past the 10 minutes.

Be sure that you plan ahead and schedule your time for exercise. When others want to schedule something else for that time, tell them you have an important meeting! What else is more important than meeting with yourself for some exercise? Lay out your exercise clothes for the next day in a place where you can see them. If you're an early morning exerciser, put your workout gear right next to the bed so that you literally have to trip over it when you get up.

Not Enough Time

So many of us live busy lives and feel that there's barely enough time for work, family life and sleep, much less exercise. But if you truly want to lose weight and get in shape, you have to set aside about an hour a day, even if broken up into segments, and make exercise as much a priority as everything else in your life. There are no quick fixes and no miracle exercise machines that will allow you to lose weight in minutes a day. Time is your best friend!

One of the best things you can do is schedule your exercise in the morning. Studies have frequently shown that morning exercisers are as much as three times more likely to consistently exercise than those who exercise at night. You get up, you exercise, and it's done for the day. Your morning, before work, school and other responsibilities, is possibly the most controllable time of your day. As the day progresses there are delays, distractions, errands, schedules and countless interruptions that may chip away at your time, and we all know that exercise is the first thing to give when we have a schedule conflict. (Morning exercise also revs up your metabolism for your day and helps burn some extra calories.)

Psychologist Dave Junno has these suggestions on how to find the time to exercise:

> Look at what you spend your time on now: are there things that actually make your efforts at dieting less successful that you could eliminate? For example, what about shaving off some couch potato time in front of the TV and devote that time to menu planning for the week or doing a physical activity. If you eat out a great deal, think about spending one hour a week meal planning and one hour a week shopping for those meals. These two hours will result in big time and money savings over the course of a week. If you have a lot of people putting demands on your time, maybe you can delegate tasks to others or let people know you are no longer available to do certain things. Sit down with a friend and brainstorm your schedule and the demands on you. Others can often see areas of potential flexibility we do not.

KEEPING ACTIVE: THE BASICS
Ways to Increase Activity Levels

Try walking sometimes instead of driving. Walk to a local shop or to a friend's house. I have a friend who loves to get espresso every weekend, but she has made a deal with herself that she needs to walk a mile to get it and a mile back. She walks more than 100 miles a year just for her espresso!

One of my silly but effective tricks is that I do some exercise every time I make a cup of tea. I like to drink several cups of herbal or green tea during the day. I work at home, so that 5 minutes it takes for the kettle to boil is exercise time for me. I do stretching and flexibility exercises, a few quick push-ups, some lunges and squats, and pretty quickly the water is boiling. Those little breaks add up to 15 minutes every workday, which adds up to an additional 75 minutes of exercising every week! Some people suggest that you do the same thing during adverts while you're watching television. Pop down on the floor and do some sit-ups, leg lifts and stretches. Keep some hand weights nearby and do bicep curls. Since there is an average of 8 minutes of adverts for every 30 minutes of television, if you watch 2 hours of television, you could end up doing a half-hour of exercise. And there's almost no activity that you can't do for 2 minutes at a time!

Speaking of television, get away from it! The amount of time you spend in front of the telly is directly related to weight gain and mindless eating! If there's something on you just can't miss, and you have home exercise equipment like a treadmill, stair-stepping machine or exercise bike, make a strict deal with yourself that you can watch your favourite programmes only if you're working out while they're on. This is a great way to get your telly fix and a workout, too!

THE IMPORTANCE OF MUSCLE

If you only have the energy or time to do one type of exercise, which should you choose – weight-bearing/strength-training or aerobics? Well, ideally, you should be doing both, but I posed this question to exercise expert Paige Waehner, who had this to say:

> I would probably choose strength training. When you build lean muscle, you're giving your body the ability to burn more calories even when you're not exercising. A pound of fat only burns around 6–10 calories each day, while a pound of muscle can burn up to 60 calories per day. Adding more muscle means burning more calories. Some strength-training workouts will also have cardiovascular benefits as well.

Waehner emphasizes an important point: Muscle is much more metaboli-cally active than fat and, as a result, a pound of muscle burns far more calo-ries than the same pound of fat. Around 60 to 75 per cent of your daily energy expenditure is accounted for by your resting metabolic rate – the calories your body uses just to keep you alive, though inactive. Even if you are in bed all day, the higher your percentage of body fat, the lower your resting metabolic rate – you'll need *fewer* calories per pound to maintain a stable weight.

In one study, after just 12 weeks, people who increased their muscle mass by 3 pounds could eat 15 per cent more calories – that's a total of 225 calories a day if you normally eat 1,500 calories a day – without gaining weight. And the people studied still lost 4 pounds of fat on average.

And remember, fat takes up a lot more space than muscle, which is far denser. Typically, in middle age, most of us trade as much as 1 pound of muscle for up to 2 pounds of fat every year – the reason for the much-lamented 'middle-age spread' in both men and women. You can lose 10 pounds of fat, gain 10 pounds of muscle and still be fitter, leaner and look far slimmer but weigh in at exactly the same weight! So don't become too scales-obsessed!

One study found that after the menopause women can reduce body fat, increase muscle mass and strengthen bones by regularly lifting moderately heavy weights. Another research study followed 24 women through a 6-month programme of periodized resistance training – that is, regularly vary-ing exercises and the order in which they're done, varying the weight used and the number of repetitions, and varying exercise frequency. This helps avoid plateaux. The women on this programme lost 7 per cent of their body fat – double the results of those doing a non-periodized routine.

Fitness and nutrition experts Ric Rooney and Bart Hanks of the Physique Transformation website (see Appendix A) recommend that men should concentrate on upper body work and women on lower body work for strength training:

> On average, a man's exercise programme works five times above the waist (chest, shoulders, back, biceps, triceps) for every time below the waist (legs). A woman's programme should do just the opposite and work five times below the waist (quads, hamstrings, calves, hips, glutes) for every time above the waist ... If squats are the king of exercises for men, lunges should be the queen of exercises for women. Lunges are a great compound movement that work the glutes, hamstrings and, to a smaller extent, the quads, all in one exercise.

A STARTER STRENGTH CIRCUIT

You can get strength-training videos and books, buy a set of hand weights or free weights, work out with resistance bands and tubes, join a gym, or get a personal trainer – there are many ways to start strength training. I really like working out with my resistance bands and hand weights.

If you want to start training at home, here is a very simple but effective approach to get you started. All you need is a circuit (series) of three exercises: lunges, push-ups and leg raises. They target the key parts of the body. Your objective is to do the exercises in a circuit, meaning that you do as many of one exercise as you can until you can't do another one, then move on to the next exercise, and so on. When you've finished one circuit, rest a minute or two, then go back through the circuit again. The objective is to repeat the circuit three times.

As you begin, keep in mind that you may only be able to do one or two of each exercise in each round of the circuit. That's fine. Rest a minute or two. Do a second circuit. Rest again, stop, or do a third circuit. Next time, see if you can add one repetition to each exercise. The point is to keep challenging yourself and to keep improving from where you began. It doesn't matter if your friend can do 10 lunges and you can only do 5. Just do what you can and try to improve on your personal best each time.

Lunges

Lunges are good for strengthening and firming your legs and bottom.

1. **Stand with your feet shoulder-width apart, keeping your hands at your sides.**
2. **Take a deep breath and step backwards with the right foot so that your right knee is a few inches above the floor. Make sure your right knee does not extend in front of/beyond the toes of your left foot. Keep your hands at your sides and look straight ahead.**
3. **Exhale and bring the right leg back to the starting position, standing with your feet apart, hands at your sides.**
4. **Repeat again with the right leg as many times as you can.**
5. **Then do the same with your left leg, repeating as many times as you can.**

Periodically, switch your lunges to forward/walking lunges:

1. Stand with your feet hip-distance apart.
2. Take a long step forwards with your right foot.
3. Bend both knees, making sure your knees and toes face forward.
4. Lower your left knee as far as you comfortably can towards the floor.
5. Return to starting position, standing straight up, and repeat with your left leg.
6. Alternate right and left legs, repeating as many times as you can.

Note: With both types of lunges, as you get stronger, you can use hand weights to increase resistance.

Once complete, move on quickly to push-ups.

Push-ups

Push-ups help strengthen your upper arms, shoulders and back.

1. Lie face down and put your hands on the floor, palms facing down, a bit more than shoulder-width apart.
2. If you are doing a full push-up, your toes should be on the floor, with your back and legs straight.
3. If a full push-up is too hard, do an easier push-up, with your knees rather than your feet/toes on the floor.
4. Exhale as you slowly push your body away from the floor using your arms.
5. Inhale while you lower your body almost to the ground, but do not touch the ground.
6. Do this as many times as you can.

Once complete, move on quickly to leg raises.

Leg Raises/Crunches

1. Lie on your back on a towel, mat or carpet. Keep your legs straight and feel your lower back pressing into the floor.
2. As you exhale, bring your knees towards your chest and raise your head off the floor. Do not curl your neck and do not try to touch your chin to your

chest. Instead, keep your lower back glued to the floor and pick a point on the ceiling. Imagine your forehead being lifted towards that point.

3. Inhale while lowering your head and straightening your legs, but do not touch the floor with your legs.
4. Repeat this as many times as you can.

Rest for 1 to 3 minutes. Then repeat the circuit, starting again with the lunges.

Sounds easy, right? Try it! After my first day's effort of two circuits (when I started, each circuit involved 5 lunges on each leg, 8 push-ups and about 15 of the leg raises/crunches), I was one hurting girl. This programme worked out muscles I didn't even know I had! I felt it for days. So get started, but go slow and don't overdo it at first.

AEROBIC/CARDIOVASCULAR EXERCISE

Aerobic exercise not only helps your heart but can burn fat and boost your resting metabolism for several hours afterward, as your muscles burn calories to recover and repair themselves. The key to getting the most benefit out of aerobics is ultimately being able to work at the right intensity for you. Your target heart rate is the pulse rate you should exercise at for maximum cardiovascular benefits. Your objective should be a minimum of 30 minutes at your target heart rate at least three times a week. Your target heart rate – the rate at which you'll burn fat – is easy to calculate. It's 220 minus your age multiplied by 0.75. Here are some examples:

Starting Rate	Age	=	x 0.75
220	25	195	146
220	30	190	143
220	40	180	135
220	50	170	128
220	60	160	120
220	70	150	113

So if you are 40 years old, your target heart rate is 200 minus 40, or 180, multiplied by 0.75, for a total of 135.

Keep in mind that this number is a goal. It's not where you're going to start out if you're just getting back into exercising.

There are many activities that are considered aerobic; which one you do depends entirely on your own preference and capabilities. You can cycle, indoors or out, on a regular or stationary bike. Swim or do water workouts. Walk outside or on a treadmill. Use a stair-stepping machine or climb stairs at your home or office. Row. Skip rope. Take an aerobics class or do an aerobics video. You can do low-impact (like an elliptical machine) or high-impact (like jogging).

WALKING: THE SUPER EXERCISE

If you have to pick one cardiovascular exercise to get started, it should be walking. One study in the *Journal of the American Medical Association* found that women who want to lose a lot of weight should walk briskly for an hour a day while cutting calories. Researchers followed 184 sedentary women who weighed an average of 200 pounds (14 st 4). The women, aged 21 to 45, were told to consume 1,200 to 1,500 calories a day and exercise 5 days a week for a year, either continuously or in 10-minute bursts. The form of exercise used was brisk walking. After a year, here's what happened:

- **The women who were walking from 50 to 60 minutes a day (either continually or in 10-minute increments) and eating 1,500 calories a day lost and kept off from 12 to 14 per cent of their starting weight, or about 25 to 30 pounds. They were burning 2,000 calories or more a week with exercise.**
- **Those who were exercising 30 to 40 minutes a day and eating around 1,500 calories lost and kept off around 9 per cent of their starting weight, or about 16 to 20 pounds. They were burning about 1,000 to 1,500 calories a week with exercise.**

Remember, this is brisk walking, not strolling through the shopping mall. If you were on a treadmill, the speed would probably be in the 3 to 4 mph range, minimum.

Speaking of treadmills, this is my favourite way of walking. I put the telly on, slap in a DVD, or pop on my headphones and pass the time while I get my aerobic exercise. And I'm not alone – treadmills are one of the most popular exercise machines at fitness clubs and at home.

But with treadmill walking it's easy to get lazy, so you need to vary the routine. One of the most effective things you can do to burn fat is raise the incline! If you raise the incline, you can burn as much as 50 per cent more calories. One simple way is to alternate 5 minutes of level walking with 5 minutes of incline and so on. Start with a small incline (e.g. 1 per cent) at the same speed, then gradually raise it. Or if your treadmill has a setting for going up and down hills, programme that setting.

Whether it's on a treadmill or outside, if you're going to get started with walking, go slow and have a plan. Beginners can start with 10 minutes of walking. Start with 2 minutes of slow walking to warm up, then go to 6 minutes at a brisker pace – that would be 3.2 to 3.7 mph on a treadmill – then cool down for 2 minutes at 2.5 to 3.2 mph.

When you're ready to take on a bit more, go to 30 minutes of walking. Start with a 5-minute warm-up, going 2.5 to 3.2 mph. Then go for 20 minutes at 3.2 to 3.7 mph. Then have a 5-minute cool-down at 2.5 to 3.2 mph.

As you get stronger, you can start adding periods of incline to this work-out (or if you're outside, head for some hills) or switch to one of the interval approaches to make it more challenging.

STRETCHING AND FLEXIBILITY

Stretching and flexibility exercises are equally important for muscle building and aerobics, because these exercises relax you, make you feel great and keep your muscles and joints in good condition. You can get a stretching tape, take a stretching class, or just follow some simple stretching programmes.

There are several types of exercises – including yoga, Pilates, water aerobics and water weight training – that I particularly recommend for thyroid patients because they combine a variety of stretching, flexibility, stress reduction and even cardiovascular benefits. Other stretching and flexibility approaches you may want to look at include some of the movement and martial arts from Asia, such as aikido, karate, tae kwon do and the softer practice tai chi, which features graceful movements designed to harmonize energy in the body.

I particularly like Pilates, because it helps build muscle, raises metabolism, relieves aching joints and muscles and can be done even by people who don't have a high level of fitness or energy. (In short, it's perfect for thyroid patients!) Pilates (pronounced p'-LAH-teez) is a method of exercise developed in the 1920s that focuses on strengthening what its founder called 'the powerhouse' – the abdomen, lower back and buttocks – that supports your body, allowing for easier movement. When starting, it's best to have a trained teacher, but some basic Pilates moves can be learned on your own. In Pilates, more isn't better. You're not pushed to do rep after rep. Instead, it encourages fewer, more precise movements performed with proper control and good form.

I started to do Pilates during the summer of 2002, and have stuck with it regularly for at least 2 hours a week. In more than 40 years of life as a non-athlete, this is the first time I've stuck to a particular exercise programme regularly for this long. It combines many of the things I love about yoga, with even more muscle building and control. I love it. I spent years with shoulder and back pain, especially that awful stabbing neck and shoulder pain that is typical of fibromyalgia. I also had quite a bit of lower back pain and chest/rib pain (known as costochondritis). About 3 months after starting Pilates, my pain was gone ... and it hasn't come back!

Luckily, I've found an affordable personal trainer who works with a friend and me on our Pilates. In addition, I purchased Mari Winsor's set of Pilates videos, which my trainer recommended. I love the 20-minute Winsor Pilates workout tape. Even on busy days, it's hard to find an excuse not to pop down on the floor and do 20 minutes, which flies by! And the more intense Winsor Pilates Accelerated Body Sculpting workout tape gives me something to aspire to, as I slowly get better at doing the exercises. I think I've found my exercise for life!

Trained doctor and fitness expert Silvia Treves – who also happens to be my Pilates trainer – has some thoughts about why Pilates is a good choice for people who may not be particularly physically fit:

> Pilates doesn't put any pressure on your joints. It gives you strength, particularly in the core area of the abdomen and lower back. At the same time, it builds flexibility. With proper instruction, there is no strain to the back and neck, and many people find that regular practice of Pilates actually resolves

chronic back and neck pain. Pilates is also a gentle way to ease into exercising. You can convert some fat to muscle, build endurance – and you can always modify the Pilates exercises to accommodate your own capabilities – so it's a good way to start off.

A SPECIAL NOTE FOR WOMEN WHO ARE STILL MENSTRUATING

Researchers have found that exercising later in your menstrual phase may help you burn more fat and feel less tired during your workout. Exercise may feel easier and your performance may actually improve during the later part of the menstrual cycle (the time between ovulation and the start of your menstrual period). During this time, the levels of oestrogen and proges-terone are highest. These hormones promote the body's use of fat as an energy supply during exercise, which helps you burn off more fat. Since the use of fat is more efficient, fewer waste products that cause exercise fatigue are produced.

So when you have more energy during the second half of your cycle, use it. You can push yourself harder during that part of the month, because you'll have more energy and get more results from your workouts. You may want to focus more on yoga, Pilates and strength training during the first half of your cycle, and emphasize higher-intensity exercise during the second half.

PART 4

The Thyroid Diet

CHAPTER 9

Your Thyroid
Diet Plans

Usually we feel that there's a large problem
and we have to fix it. The instruction is to stop.
Do something unfamiliar. Do anything besides
rushing off in the same old direction, up to the
same old tricks.

– PEMA CHÖDRÖN

When you're dealing with a metabolic issue like thyroid disease, as well as many possible impediments to weight loss, finding a successful approach that will work for you is part science, part instinct. You and your body *know* how to lose weight; it's just a matter of trying out the likeliest approaches, observing your body's responses and monitoring how you feel until you find an approach that works, then tweaking it so that it fits you.

We all know people who stay slender and don't vary in weight and, let's face it, we feel green with envy about them sometimes. But if you're really honest about it, except for the rare freak of nature or teenage athletes with supercharged metabolisms, you will rarely see them wolfing down everything in sight and loading up on junk food. They've most likely come up with a way of eating that works for them, and they are usually physically active in some way. My husband is one of these people. At 6'3", with a body mass index around 22, he's quite trim. His cholesterol is around 160. His blood pressure is 105/60. I don't think he's varied 5 pounds since I met him. People look at him and say, 'Oh, you can eat anything you want and not put on weight,' or 'You have such a good metabolism – you're so lucky.'

But that's not the case. Yes, he's fortunate in that he doesn't appear to have any major metabolic impediments – like a thyroid condition – that make it easier to gain weight. But he has also never abused his metabolism (by smoking, or crash dieting, or not eating regularly, or bingeing on junk food) and he has listened to his body and figured out what it needs. He eats to live rather than lives to eat. He doesn't vary much in what and how he eats. He always has to have a protein, a starch and fruit for breakfast. He always has veggies or a salad for lunch, with a sandwich. Dinner is a protein, a starch, a salad and a green vegetable. (If I haven't made a vegetable, he'll add raw broccoli to his salad.) At night, his snack never varies – an apple and some peanuts. I tallied it all up one day and he gets at least 3 servings of fruit and 4 servings of vegetables every day, minimum. And he drinks water all day long – with breakfast, lunch, dinner, his snack, and throughout the day. He doesn't use mayonnaise or salad dressings, rarely eats sweets, and I think I've seen him have a fizzy drink a half-dozen times in 10 years. He drinks alcohol occasionally, but not often. On top of that, he does a bit of walking every day, to and from work, and weekly Pilates sessions, plus some gardening – but he's far from an exercise hound. When we've been on holiday or out for a special night and he's eaten more treats or junk food than usual, he immediately gets back on track, returning to his usual way of eating.

The key for him is *consistency*. Almost every day he eats well, in a way that allows him to maintain a healthy weight. And when he has a treat here and there, he just gets back on the programme the next day. He's following what some people call the 90/10 rule of weight management – he maintains healthy eating habits and activity at least 90 per cent of the time, then can splurge 10 per cent of the time.

My husband is not a metabolic miracle; nor is he luckier than anyone else! He simply has found the precise formula that takes care of his body in the best way possible. Your job is to find the system that is going to work best for you.

THE PLANS

I have not set out one specific plan and presented it as the plan that will work for you and everyone else with a thyroid problem, because I've discovered that there simply isn't one plan that will work for everyone. Some thyroid patients are carbohydrate sensitive and find that they can only lose weight when strictly limiting starchy foods. You could just as easily be a thyroid patient who actually gains weight on the low-carb Atkins approach! Or you may be more calorie sensitive and find that you only lose weight when you take your calorie levels lower. Or you may need a very balanced approach of proteins, starches, vegetables, fruits, fat and so forth.

If all this sounds confusing, relax, because I've outlined a number of approaches that you can try. Your objective is to find the plan that works best with your unique metabolism.

WHICH PLAN IS RIGHT FOR YOU?

Complete the following checklists to help determine which one of the plans is the best starting point for you.

❏ You have tried one of the low-carb diets like Atkins, and you gained weight while following it.

❏ You truly enjoy eating vegetables and fruits.

❏ You feel your best after a meal that contains protein, starch and some vegetables or fruit.

❏ You need variety in your diet.

If you've ticked two or more of the above statements, then you should start with the Free-Form Plan.

❑ You frequently crave things like pasta, bread, rice, potatoes and sweet puddings.

❑ Once you get started eating things like pasta, bread, rice, potatoes and sweet puddings, you find it hard to stop.

❑ After you eat things like pasta, bread, rice, potatoes and sweet puddings, you find yourself feeling hungry again fairly quickly.

❑ You find that after you eat a piece of cake or a bowl of pasta, you temporarily end up a pound or two heavier on the scales the next day.

If you've ticked two or more of the above statements, then it's likely that carbohydrates are a problem for you. You should start with the Carb-Sensitive Plan.

❑ You have tried a diet like Weight Watchers and gained weight while following it.

❑ You have tried a low-carb diet like Atkins and gained weight while following it.

❑ You suspect that you probably eat too much, but you don't keep track.

❑ You find that you can gain weight on what others would consider cutting back or a diet.

If you've ticked two or more of the above statements, then you should start with the Calorie-Sensitive Plan.

If you found yourself agreeing with many of the statements in all of the categories, then start out with the Free-Form Plan.

While the checklists can help you choose a plan to start with, read through all the plan guidelines. You will probably have an instinctual sense of which plan may be the best for you to try first. If you really listen, you know your body better than you think.

Foods, some suggested menus and a variety of tasty, healthful recipes are featured in Chapter 10. You'll find that those guidelines will help you follow the plan of your choice more easily.

Follow the plan suggested by your checklists, or try whichever plan makes the most sense for you. Give it at least 4 weeks. I mean it – 4 weeks. I know the temptation is to try it for 4 days and, if you don't notice the scales going down, you'll abandon it for the next plan. But give it 4 weeks. See how you do. Note how you feel. Keep a food journal and track types of foods, carbohydrate intake, fat (including saturated fat), your moods, exercise level, menstrual periods, water, supplements and daily weight so that you can see how you're doing and what might be affecting your weight.

After 4 weeks, if you've lost a few pounds (and remember, when you're dealing with a thyroid problem, consider it a resounding success if you have lost 1 pound in a week!) you'll want to stick with the plan you're on. But go back and look at the notes you've kept. Did you find that you didn't have any weight loss on the days after you ate dairy, or you even bloated up and gained a bit? Think about cutting down on dairy as you move forward. Did you notice that if you met your water goals one day, the next day you saw some weight loss on the scales? This tells you that you really need to keep your water level high. In contrast, if you felt terrible quite a bit of the time, or haven't lost anything or even gained weight, then try one of the other plans. And give that plan 4 weeks.

I'm not offering a quick fix. If there were a miracle diet, you and I wouldn't need to be here. It usually takes quite a bit of time to become hypothyroid and for metabolism to get off track. It can take just as much time or more to get your thyroid back towards balance and help re-energize your metabolism so that you start losing weight. And once you're hypothyroid, you're likely to remain that way, so we're looking for a way of eating that is going to work for life.

But have faith. You *will* find that one of the following plans contains an approach that will work for you!

THE FREE-FORM PLAN

The free-form plan is straightforward and gives you quite a bit of leeway. It's a balanced, healthy starting point. If you already know you are extremely carbohydrate sensitive, this may not be the place to start, but if you're not sure, this is a good plan to follow.

- Eat 3 meals a day.
- Protein – each meal should include 1–2 portions of lean protein.
- Low-glycaemic vegetables – eat all you want and make sure you're getting at least 6 servings a day.
- Low-glycaemic fruits – 1–2 servings a day maximum.
- Low-glycaemic starches – 2–3 servings a day maximum.
- Good fat – a small serving with each meal and snack.
- Snacks – 1–2 per day if needed (but avoid eating after 8 p.m.).
- Treats – very sparingly; maybe a small serving once or twice a week at most.
- Water – 2 litres, minimum.
- Supplements – your choice as per your practitioner's recommendation.
- Fibre – 25 grams, minimum.

You don't need to count calories with this diet – focusing on lean proteins, plenty of vegetables, good fats and limited starches and fruits naturally keeps the calories at a healthy level.

FREEFORM PLAN DAILY CHECKLISTS

Date: **Morning Weight:**

Breakfast   **Lunch**   **Dinner**
Protein ☐   Fat ☐   Protein ☐   Fat ☐   Protein ☐   Fat ☐

Vegetables: 6 servings
☐   ☐   ☐   ☐   ☐   ☐

Fruits: 1–2 Servings   Low-Glycaemic Starches: 2–3 Servings
☐   ☐   ☐   ☐   ☐

Optional Snack 1 ☐   Optional Snack 2 ☐   Treat? ☐

Water: cross off as you go (ml):   500   500   500   500

Fibre: cross off as you go (grams):   5   5   5   5   5

Exercise:

Supplements:

Notes:

FREEFORM PLAN DAILY CHECKLISTS

Date: **Morning Weight:**

Breakfast   **Lunch**   **Dinner**
Protein ☐   Fat ☐   Protein ☐   Fat ☐   Protein ☐   Fat ☐

Vegetables: 6 servings

☐   ☐   ☐   ☐   ☐   ☐

Fruits: 1–2 Servings   Low-Glycaemic Starches: 2–3 Servings

☐   ☐   ☐   ☐   ☐

Optional Snack 1 ☐   Optional Snack 2 ☐   Treat? ☐

Water: cross off as you go (ml):   500   500   500   500

Fibre: cross off as you go (grams):   5   5   5   5   5

Exercise:

Supplements:

Notes:

CARB-SENSITIVE PLAN

- Eat 3 meals a day.
- Protein – each meal should include 1–2 portions of lean protein.
- Low-glycaemic vegetables – eat all you want and make sure you're getting at least 6 servings a day.
- Low-glycaemic fruits – 1 serving a day.
- Low-glycaemic starches – 1–2 servings a day.
- Good fat – a small serving with each meal and snack.
- Snacks – 1–2 per day if needed (but avoid eating after 8 p.m.).
- Treats – very sparingly; maybe a small serving once or twice a week at most (and avoid carbohydrate treats).
- Water – 2 litres, minimum.
- Supplements – your choice as per your practitioner's recommendation.
- Fibre – 30 grams, minimum.

While you don't want to go overboard calorie-wise on the carb-sensitive plan, you don't have to be particularly concerned about calories. One pilot study followed three groups: one on a low-fat controlled-calorie diet, the second on a low-carbohydrate diet at the same calorie levels, and the third on a low-carbohydrate diet at 300 more calories per day. Statistically, all the groups lost about the same amount of weight, despite the fact that the third group technically should have lost 7 pounds less than the other groups, if you follow the 3,500 calories equals 1 pound dictum.

CARBOHYDRATE-SENSITIVE PLAN DAILY CHECKLISTS

Date: **Morning Weight:**

Breakfast   **Lunch**   **Dinner**
Protein ☐   Fat ☐   Protein ☐   Fat ☐   Protein ☐   Fat ☐

Vegetables: 6 servings

☐   ☐   ☐   ☐   ☐   ☐

Fruits: 1 Serving   Low-Glycaemic Starches: 1–2 Servings

☐   ☐   ☐

Optional Snack 1 ☐   Optional Snack 2 ☐   Treat? ☐

Water: cross off as you go (ml):   500   500   500   500

Fibre: cross off as you go (grams):   5   5   5   5   5   5

Exercise:

Supplements:

Notes:

CARBOHYDRATE-SENSITIVE PLAN DAILY CHECKLISTS

Date: **Morning Weight:**

Breakfast   **Lunch**   **Dinner**
Protein ☐   Fat ☐   Protein ☐   Fat ☐   Protein ☐   Fat ☐

Vegetables: 6 servings
☐   ☐   ☐   ☐   ☐   ☐

Fruits: 1 Serving   Low-Glycaemic Starches: 1–2 Servings
☐   ☐   ☐

Optional Snack 1 ☐   Optional Snack 2 ☐   Treat? ☐

Water: cross off as you go (ml):   500   500   500   500

Fibre: cross off as you go (grams):   5   5   5   5   5   5

Exercise:

Supplements:

Notes:

THE CALORIE-SENSITIVE PLAN

Some people simply can't lose weight without cutting calories. With the calorie-sensitive plan, you'll need to do more tracking of foods, so you may want to invest in one of the computer programmes or tools – like Diet Power or the Personal Food Analyst – that will help you keep track of your intake fairly closely.

Your aim is to stay within your calorie target, getting approximately 35 per cent of your calories from lean protein, 20 per cent from low-glycaemic vegetables, 15 per cent from low-glycaemic fruits and starches, and 30 per cent from good fats.

How Many Calories Do You Need?

The number of calories you need should take into account height, weight and age. One way to calculate your basal metabolic rate (BMR) caloric intake is with the Harris-Benedict equation, which differs for men and women:

Men:
BMR= 66 + (13.7 x weight in kilograms) + (5 x height in centimetres) – (6.8 x age in years)

Women:
BMR = 655 + (9.6 x weight in kilograms) + (1.8 x height in centimetres) – (4.7 x age in years)

Note: To calculate your weight in kilograms, multiply your divide your weight in pounds by 2.2 (to convert from stones to pounds, remember that each stone equals 14 pounds). To calculate your height in centimetres, multiply your height in inches by 2.54.

Here's how it works for a 14 st 4 person who is 5'8" and 45 years old.

14 st 4 is 200 pounds
200 pounds is 90.9 kilograms (200 ÷ by 2.2)
68 inches is 172.72 centimetres (68 x 2.54)
Age 45

Man, 200 pounds, 5'8"

66+	(13.7 x wt in kg)	+ (5 x ht in cm)	– (6.8 x age in yrs)
66+	(13.7 x 90.9)	+ (5 x 172.72)	– (6.8 x 45)
66+	1245.5	+ 863.6	+ 306.0
=	**1,869 calories**		

Woman, 200 pounds, 5'8"

655+	(9.6 x wt in kg)	+ (1.8 x ht in cm)	– (4.7 x age in yrs)
655+	(9.6 x 90.0)	+ (1.8 x 172.82)	– (4.7 x 45)
655+	872.7	+ 310.9	– 211.5
=	**1,627 calories**		

Unless you are unusually active, meaning you work out at least 1 hour four times a week or more, this level of calories should be your target level. (If you do work out more than this, multiply the calorie level by a factor of 1.3 to take into account your workouts.) If you don't see any weight loss within 2 weeks, try cutting another 150 calories and see if that triggers weight loss over a 2-week period.

MEN'S CALORIE WORKSHEET

Men: How Many Calories Do You Need?

Basal Metabolic Rate = 66 + (13.7 x wt in kg) + (5 x ht in cm) – (6.8 x age in yr)

Your Weight in Pounds   _____

Divide by 2.2   _____

= Your Weight in Kilograms   _____

Your Height in Inches   _____

Multiplied by 2.54   _____

= Your Height in Centimetres   _____

Your Age in Years   _____

                                                                66

                                                                +

13.7 x   _____   =   _____

                    (your weight

                    in kilograms)   +

5 x   _____   =   _____

                    (your height

                    in centimetres) +

Subtotal   _____

                                                       –

6.8 x   _____   =   _____

                    (your age

                    in years)

Total   _____

WOMEN'S CALORIE WORKSHEET

Women – How Many Calories Do You Need?

Basal Metabolic Rate = 655 + (9.6 x wt in kg) + (1.8 x ht in cm) – (4.7 x age in yr)

Your Weight in Pounds _____

Divide by 2.2 _____

= Your Weight in Kilograms _____

Your Height in Inches _____

Multiplied by 2.54 _____

= Your Height in Centimetres _____

Your Age in Years _____

65.5
+
_____

9.6 x _____ =

(your weight

in kilograms) +

1.8 x _____ = _____

(your height

in centimetres) +

Subtotal _____

–

4.7 x _____ = _____

(your age

in years)

Total _____

CALORIE-SENSITIVE PLAN DAILY CHECKLISTS

Date: **Morning Weight:**

Breakfast calories: _____   **Lunch calories:** _____   **Dinner calories:** _____

Snacks/calories:

Water: cross off as you go (ml):   500   500   500   500

Fibre: cross off as you go (grams):   5   5   5   5   5   5

Exercise:

Supplements:

Notes:

Date: **Morning Weight:**

Breakfast calories: _____   **Lunch calories:** _____   **Dinner calories:** _____

Snacks/calories:

Water: cross off as you go (ml):   500   500   500   500

Fibre: cross off as you go (grams):   5   5   5   5   5   5

Exercise:

Supplements:

Notes:

TWEAKING YOUR MEALS AND FOODS

One of the key ways you'll be working with your diet is to tweak your plan to make sure it fits you perfectly and helps you lose weight. For example, you may find that you are losing weight, but extremely slowly. Don't abandon that plan and start a different one, hoping you'll lose pounds more quickly! If you are losing, you are on the right track. Instead, consider making some modifications to your plan to see how you respond.

Don't make all the modifications at once, however, or you won't know which change is working. After you make a modification, allow yourself at least a week before you decide to abandon it, adopt it permanently, or try another modification or plan. Some of the most helpful tweaks to your plan might be the following:

- Up the water – your body needs a constant, steady source of water in order to flush out toxins and fat and to keep metabolism functioning smoothly. So if you're drinking 2 litres a day, try adding three to five more 250-ml glasses so that you're drinking 3 litres of water. And if you're drinking more than 3 litres a day, try working your way up to drinking 30 ml for every pound of body weight.
- Cut back on starches – some people are so sensitive to starchy carbohydrates that, if they eat any, they can't lose much weight at all. Whatever plan you are on, one option is to drop one serving of starchy carbs each day to see what happens.
- On a calorie-sensitive plan, cut calories – sometimes, the difference between stalling out and losing weight is a matter of a few calories. If you're on the calorie-sensitive plan, cut 50 or 100 calories a day. It may mean the difference between losing and staying where you are.
- Drop your snacks – if you're a veteran snacker, consider dropping your snacks. Try focusing on eating a larger breakfast and a slightly larger lunch.

IMPLEMENTING YOUR PLAN
What Is Your Optimal Weight?

I can't tell you at which weight you'll feel the best, and there are many different expert opinions. One of the simplest formulas is this: for women, allow 100 pounds for the first 5 feet (1.5 metres) and 5 pounds for each additional inch (2.5 cm); for men, allow 110 pounds for the first 5 feet and 5 pounds for each additional inch. More sophisticated charts differentiate between frame size, by gender and height.

Women				Men			
Height	Small Frame	Medium Frame	Large Frame	Height	Small Frame	Medium Frame	Large Frame
4'10"	102–111	109–121	118–131	5'2"	128–134	131–141	138–150
4'11"	103–113	111–123	120–134	5'3"	130–136	133–143	140–153
5'0"	104–115	113–126	122–137	5'4"	132–138	135–145	142–156
5'1"	106–118	115–129	125–140	5'5"	134–140	137–148	144–160
5'2"	108–121	118–132	128–143	5'6"	136–142	139–151	146–164
5'3"	111–124	121–135	131–147	5'7"	138–145	142–154	149–168
5'4"	114–127	124–138	134–151	5'8"	140–148	145–157	152–172
5'5"	117–130	127–141	137–155	5'9"	142–151	148–160	155–176
5'6"	120–133	130–144	140–159	5'10"	144–154	151–163	158–180
5'7"	123–136	133–147	143–163	5'11"	146–157	154–166	161–184
5'8"	126–139	136–150	146–167	6'0"	149–160	157–170	164–188
5'9"	129–142	139–153	149–170	6'1"	152–164	160–174	168–192
5'10"	132–145	142–156	152–173	6'2"	155–168	164–178	172–197
5'11"	135–148	145–159	155–176	6'3"	158–172	167–182	176–202
6'0"	138–151	148–162	158–179	6'4"	162–176	171–187	181–207

Ultimately, I know you have a number in your mind. It may be based on the above charts and calculations. More likely, it is based on a weight at which you've felt and looked your best in the past. Now, I want you to put that number in the back of your mind. It may be your final goal, but you need to set realistic goals along the way.

Body Mass Index

To set your initial goals, you need to know your body mass index (BMI). A rough calculation of your BMI is your weight in pounds divided by your height in inches squared (lb/in²) multiplied by 703. Here's an example:

Suppose you are 5'8" and weigh 200 pounds (14 st 4).

There are 12 inches in a foot, so 5 feet in inches is 5 x 12, or 60. Since you're 5'8", we need to add 8 inches, so your height in inches is 68.

68 squared (68 x 68) equals 4,624.

Take your weight, 200 and divide it by 4,624.

That's 0.0432525951557093.

Now multiply by 703.

That equals 30.4065743944637.

So, rounded off, your body mass index would be 30.4.

BODY MASS INDEX CHART

Healthy weight BMI	18.5–25
Overweight BMI	26–30
Obese BMI	31–40
Morbidly obese BMI	Above 40

In our example, a 200-pound person (14 st 4) who is 5'8" with a BMI of 30.4 would be considered overweight.

In addition to the calculation method, the following BMI table can help you. There are also numerous online calculators where you enter your height and weight and your BMI is calculated. I have one on my site at http://www.goodmetabolism.com.

BODY MASS INDEX (BMI) FOR ADULTS

BMI Height (in inches)	Healthy range						Overweight					Obese					
	19	20	21	22	23	24	25	26	27	28	29	30	31	32	33	34	35
									Weight (in pounds)								
4'10" (58")	91	96	100	105	110	115	119	124	129	134	138	143	148	153	158	162	167
4'11" (59")	94	99	104	109	114	119	124	128	133	138	143	148	153	158	163	168	173
5' (60")	97	102	107	112	118	123	128	133	138	143	148	153	158	163	168	174	179
5'1" (61")	100	106	111	116	122	127	132	137	143	148	153	158	164	169	174	180	185
5'2" (62")	104	109	115	120	126	131	136	142	147	153	158	164	169	175	180	186	191
5'3" (63")	107	113	118	124	130	135	141	146	152	158	163	169	175	180	186	191	197
5'4" (64")	110	116	122	128	134	140	145	151	157	163	169	174	180	186	192	197	204
5'5" (65")	114	120	126	132	138	144	150	156	162	168	174	180	186	192	198	204	210
5'6" (66")	118	124	130	136	142	148	155	161	167	173	179	186	192	198	204	210	216
5'7" (67")	121	127	134	140	146	153	159	166	172	178	185	191	198	204	211	217	223
5'8" (68")	125	131	138	144	151	158	164	171	177	184	190	197	203	210	216	223	230
5'9" (69")	128	135	142	149	155	162	169	176	182	189	196	203	209	216	223	230	236
5'10" (70")	132	139	146	153	160	167	174	181	188	195	202	209	216	222	229	236	243
5'11" (71")	136	143	150	157	165	172	179	186	193	200	208	215	222	229	236	243	250
6' (72")	140	147	154	162	169	177	184	191	199	206	213	221	228	235	242	250	258
6'1" (73")	144	151	159	166	174	182	189	197	204	212	219	227	235	242	250	257	265
6'2" (74")	148	155	163	171	179	186	194	202	210	218	225	233	241	249	256	264	272
6'3" (75")	152	160	168	176	184	192	200	208	216	224	232	240	248	256	264	272	279
6'4" (76")	156	164	172	180	189	197	205	213	221	230	239	246	254	263	271	279	287

Source: Centers for Disease Control and Prevention, National Center for Chronic Disease Prevention and Health Promotion, Division of Nutrition and Physical Activity. 2003.

If you belong to a gym, work with a fitness trainer, or see a nutritional expert, they can also perform more detailed BMI calculations that take into account important fat-measurement spots. The online PhysiqueTransformation.com site has a fairly detailed online BMI calculator that tracks waist and wrist measurements in addition to height and weight if you want even more accuracy.

Excess fat in the abdominal area is a risk factor for insulin resistance and other diseases. The waist measurement at which there is a definite increase in risk is 40 inches or more for men and 35 inches or more for women.

Setting Realistic Goals

- **Phase 1/Goal 1: If you have a BMI over 30, your first goal should be to lose enough weight to get into the BMI range of 25–29. This will automatically reduce the risk of various diseases and help make your metabolism more efficient. You should also target a waist measurement reduction of 5 per cent.**
- **Phase 2/Goal 2: If you're in the 25–29 level (or you've lost enough weight in phase 1), then your goal should be to get down to a BMI of just below 25. At this point, you are no longer overweight. You have greatly reduced health risks, improved your metabolism, no doubt look like a different person and have more energy and greater fitness.**
- **Phase 3/Goal 3: If your ultimate goal weight is less than where you are with a BMI of a little less than 25, then keep working on weight loss until you reach that objective.**

In each phase, you should target a 5 per cent reduction in waist measurement. The following chart may be a help:

WAIST MEASUREMENT REDUCTION TARGETS

Waist (in inches)	Phase I 5 per cent Less	Phase II 5 per cent Less	Phase III 5 per cent Less
28	27	25	24
29	28	26	25
30	29	27	26
31	29	28	27
32	30	29	27
33	31	30	28
34	32	31	29
35	33	32	30
36	34	32	31
37	35	33	32
38	36	34	33
39	37	35	33
40	38	36	34
41	39	37	35
42	40	38	36
43	41	39	37
44	42	40	38
45	43	41	39

Let's use our previous example of a 5'8" person who is 200 pounds (14 st 4). Current BMI is 30.4. At a weight of 180 (12 st 12), the BMI would be 27. So 27 is overweight but not obese, and it's a great first goal. That would be a target weight loss of 20 pounds, or 10 per cent of body weight.

During phase 1, be realistic and assume it will take at least a week to lose a pound, so a 20-pound weight loss would probably take you at least 20 weeks, or about 5 months.

The next target should be a BMI of 24, or 160 pounds (11 st 6). That's another 20 pounds, or about 11 per cent of body weight. At this point, your metabolism may be more efficient and you are hopefully getting more activity and exercise, so weight loss could go faster – maybe 1½ pounds a week. Or it could stay at around 1 pound per week, so count on another 13 to 20 weeks, or 3 to 5 months.

At this point, you will be 160 pounds and a normal weight according to BMI. But you may still want to go a bit further. If you're a woman, you may feel that you would look your best at around 145 pounds (10 st 5) (which would be a very lean BMI of 21). So that's still another 15 pounds, or around 10 per cent of your body weight to go. Figure on another 15 weeks, or 4 months. If you're a man, you might feel like you'll look your best at 150 (10 st 10) – a BMI of 23 – in which case you only have 10 more pounds to go, or another 10 weeks. Figure on 2 to 3 months.

So within about a year, you are lean and healthy and have reached your goal! And most importantly, you have learned how to eat and exercise to stay that way!

SPECIAL GUIDELINES FOR THYROID DIETERS

No matter which plan you choose, when you are following a weight-loss programme there are some considerations you need to keep in mind that apply specifically to you as a thyroid patient.

Patience! Patience! And More Patience!

You are going to need a great deal of patience and perseverance, because even if you are doing everything right diet-wise, weight loss may go far more slowly than you would like. Celebrate your resounding success even if you lose a pound a week. Do not compare your results with anyone else's.

Although many diet programmes recommend that you diet with a buddy, this is one time when it might be better not to, unless he or she is hypothyroid, too. Because people with normal thyroid function are likely to lose weight faster than you. Not fair, but a fact of life. So keep the faith and don't let slow progress make you lose your determination to stick with the programme!

Exercise

Don't forget that you have to exercise. It's not optional. Weight-bearing/muscle-building exercise is critical to raising metabolism. And aerobic exercise helps burn calories.

Some diets and weight-loss programmes tell you that you can lose weight without exercise. That may be true for some people and some programmes. But it's not likely to be true for most thyroid patients. And what those diet programmes don't tell you is that most people who are not exercising will eventually regain the weight over time. Even if you're not a big fan of physical activity, you'll have to accept it: exercise is not optional.

Retesting

You will probably be adding fibre to your diet, so you should have your thyroid function retested about 6 to 8 weeks after you stabilize at your new level of fibre intake. You may need a change in your dosage of thyroid hormone replacement. Also, if you lose more than 10 per cent of your body weight, that is also a time to get retested to see if you need a dosage adjustment.

Mind Those Starchy Carbs!

Many thyroid patients report that they are only able to lose weight when they dramatically cut down on starchy carbohydrates – like bread, sugar, pasta, fizzy drinks and puddings – and limit carbs mainly to vegetables with some fruit. While there are thyroid patients who process carbs with no difficulty and can lose weight on a more old-fashioned food pyramid diet that emphasizes cereals, grains and bread, they seem to be the exception rather than the rule.

Keep Protein Intake Higher to Protect Hair

Hair loss is a concern for many thyroid patients, and some who start a weight-loss programme will find that hair loss increases. Frequently, this is a sign of protein deficiency. Some experts, for example, say protein intake should be as much as 0.5 grams for each pound of body weight. Try to emphasize low-fat, protein-dense food sources, like fish or lean cuts of meat and poultry.

Try One Thing at a Time

There's a tendency to want to try everything at the same time, but then it's hard to tell what is actually working. It's better to implement changes more slowly so that you can gauge what works. For example, start with dietary changes. After a few weeks, if you feel that you've found a decent way of eating, try one supplement to see if it helps speed weight loss, or curbs cravings, or reduces hypothyroid symptoms. If a particular supplement helps, you may want to try another as well. (But trying too many at the same time means you won't know which ones are really working.) Then add exercise. (Weight-bearing exercise replaces fat with muscle. Muscle takes up far less space than fat, so you may lose fat, gain muscle and show less change on the scales than you do in terms of inches lost.) Ultimately, you'll arrive at a combination of approaches that will work best for you.

Measure Regularly

Hopping on the scales to keep track of weight loss is important, but not as important as keeping track of measurements. Particularly for thyroid patients, who may have more early results in building muscle than in losing pounds, keeping track of measurements can provide important feedback and may even provide incentive on those days or weeks when you don't see much movement on the scales.

CHAPTER 10

What to Eat:
Recipes

Tell me what you eat and I will tell you what
you are.

– ANTHELME BRILLAT-SAVARIN

Now that you know about the plans and what general categories of foods
you should be eating, what specifically should you eat? This chapter looks
at the best types of foods to eat in each category, some meal ideas, serving
sizes and portions, and delicious, healthy recipes.

LEAN PROTEINS

When choosing proteins, your objective is to choose lean proteins. That
means staying away from meats that are high in saturated fats. Some of the
best proteins include:

Eggs

Low-fat milk

Low-fat cheeses

Neufchâtel cheese

Feta cheese

Fish, shellfish

Lean beef (sirloin, top round,
   tenderloin)

Beans

Lean pork (pork loin, tenderloin, boiled
   ham)

Tofu, tempeh, soy/veggie burgers

Lunch meats: fat-free or low-fat

Poultry (skinless): turkey breast
   (including minced), chicken breast,
   turkey bacon

Some of the proteins to avoid are:

- **Beef brisket, liver, ribeye steaks and other fatty cuts of beef**
- **Bacon, other fatty cuts of pork, honey-baked ham**
- **Chicken and turkey wings, legs and thighs**
- **Duck and goose**
- **Full-fat dairy products**

One of the least familiar meats to mention is buffalo, also known as bison. With an interest in lower-fat, higher-protein red meat and with increasing concerns over diseases in cows, buffalo is destined to become an attractive option. Jim McCauley, who created the recipes for this book, admits that he is a card-carrying carnivore – a true red meat lover.

> I've tried to go without, but I really miss it. I know that I can't have it every day. It's not healthy. My cholesterol would go through the roof. So I started eating bison (also known as buffalo). Why? It tastes great, it's healthier than most other meats and it satisfies my beef craving. Nutritionally, it provides more protein and nutrients with fewer calories and less fat. Because bison is a dense meat, it tends to satisfy you more with less. Bison has a few considerations – because it's so lean, it can get dry and tough if you don't cook it gently. Do not use high temperatures when cooking bison. If cooking bison stew meat, use a slow cooker. If cooking a bison roast, use a 300-degree [150°C/GM2] oven. (Due to bison's low-fat content, it cooks faster than higher fat-content meats.) It can be ordered on the Internet and shipped frozen to you. Bison comes in the same cuts as beef – mince, steaks, roasts.

Jim also loves bison burgers. He says it satisfies his hamburger craving. I didn't try bison until Jim kept recommending it. I, too, am a red meat fanatic and, lazy cook that I am, I was delighted to find that my local market has precooked bison burger patties. Two minutes in the microwave and they're ready. They're absolutely delicious, and one burger with a salad fills me up for hours.

While we're on the topic of meat, let's look at pork loin. Pork tenderloin (or loin) is lower in calories than chicken and lower in cholesterol. It's slightly higher in fat but not significantly. Pork is lower in fat, calories and cholesterol than many other meats and poultry. Any cuts from the loin – like pork chops and pork roast – are actually leaner than skinless chicken thigh, according to US Department of Agriculture data. Jim McCauley says,

> I love chicken, but there are days I just can't put another piece of chicken in my body. Won't go. Just can't do it. So, without any other changes to the recipe, substitute pork loin. Pork is quite lean and cooks the same as chicken. And you don't have to pull the skin off it like you do chicken. Less mess. Great flavour. In any recipe calling for chicken, you can substitute pork loin.

I love cooking a pork loin roast as a special Sunday dinner. It's easy (a dash of Worcestershire sauce, some garlic and a few tablespoons of olive oil and I pop it into the oven to roast, basting periodically while it's cooking.) And if you make a large enough roast, you'll have terrific leftovers for lunch or dinner next day.

Jim and I are both fans of protein in the morning. His nutritionist told him that he doesn't have to limit egg consumption (within reason) if he uses omega-3 eggs. These eggs are from regular chickens that have been fed a diet of grains high in flaxseed. As a result, they are high in alpha-linolenic acid (ALA), an omega-3 essential fatty acid that can have positive health effects. Omega-3 eggs are not genetically engineered. In studies, even eating two a day did not raise LDL cholesterol and were actually shown to raise HDL (the 'good' cholesterol) and lower triglycerides. Eggs are actually considered a near-perfect protein, because they contain a wealth of amino acids. Jim doesn't like egg-white omelets (smart guy – I don't either!), so he recommends using one omega-3 egg yolk and two portions of egg whites, which gives you a better texture and taste – and the right colour! Otherwise, you can use omega-3 eggs just as you would other eggs. They are somewhat more expensive than regular eggs, but the health advantage justifies the cost.

Jim trained at the French Culinary Institute in New York City, where he learned to cook what he calls the traditional 'heart attack on a plate' dishes filled with butter and double cream. He still loves to use cream sauces, but he frequently substitutes tinned evaporated skim milk for the cream. It's thick, rich and usually an acceptable substitution. Jim says, 'The main taste difference to me is that the evaporated milk is sweeter than the cream. I have to adjust seasonings to compensate. The savings in fat percentage of the final dish is astounding.'

Yogurt cheese is one of Jim's favourites for protein and he uses it in many recipes. It's actually a staple food in the Middle East, where it's called *lebneh*. To make yogurt cheese, get low-fat (1 per cent) plain yogurt in bulk. Get out a coffee filter (or a paper towel will do), a sieve/strainer and a bowl that is slightly larger than the sieve. Place the sieve in the bowl, line the sieve with the coffee filter (or paper towel), scoop the yogurt into the sieve and cover with plastic wrap. Place on a shelf in the refrigerator. The next morning, pour out the water that has drained from the yogurt into the bowl. You can now put the yogurt in a container. This is yogurt cheese. Jim explains, 'I use it on baked potatoes. I use it for dessert. I love having it on hand. Mixed with salsa, it's a great dip! It's an excellent substitute for soured cream/soft cream cheese.'

Some of my most memorable breakfasts have been with my fellow Middle Easterners. We have lebneh with a little olive oil drizzled over it, a handful of olives, a piece of cheese, some fresh pita bread and hot minty tea. This is usually served with a big bowl of *zaartar* for dipping. Zaartar is a blend of herbs that is popular in the Middle East. It usually includes thyme, sesame seeds and sumac bark. Sounds and looks strange, but tastes extraordinarily delicious. You dip your bread in the lebneh, then spoon on a bit of zaartar and it's delicious. (You can get zaartar at any Middle Eastern grocery or delicatessen.)

What About Beans?

Beans are a healthy, high-fibre source of protein. But keep in mind that since most beans are also very high in carbohydrates, they need to count as a combination protein/starch. If you eat a starch on top of beans, you're getting a double serving. The best beans include:

- Chickpeas
- Lima beans
- Black beans

- **Kidney beans**
- **Lentils.**

LOW-GLYCAEMIC CARBOHYDRATES

Low-glycaemic refers to the glycaemic index (GI). The GI basically is a measure of how quickly your blood sugar levels will rise after you eat a particular food. To determine a food's GI rating, portions of the food are given to people who have fasted overnight. Their blood sugar is then monitored over time and the rise in blood sugar is calculated. Foods with a lower-glycaemic index will create a slower rise in blood sugar and foods with a higher-glycaemic index will create a faster rise in blood sugar.

Low-Glycaemic Vegetables

Some of the most low-glycaemic vegetables that you can safely include in your diet include:

Artichokes	Asparagus
Aubergines	Beans and legumes
Broccoli	Brussels sprouts
Cauliflower	Celery
Courgettes	Cucumbers
Green beans	Green peppers
Lettuce	Mushrooms
Spinach	Tomatoes

The higher-glycaemic vegetables that you should limit are:

Beets	Carrots
Celery root	Corn
Parsnips	Peas
Red potatoes	Rutabaga
Sweet potatoes	Turnips
White potatoes	Winter squash
Yams	

Low-Glycaemic Fruits

Some of the most low-glycaemic fruits that you can safely include in your diet are:

Apples	Apricots
Blackberries	Blueberries
Cantaloupe melons	Cherries
Grapefruits	Nectarines
Peaches	Plums
Raspberries	Strawberries

The higher-glycaemic fruits that you should limit are:

Bananas	Grapes
Honeydew melons	Orange juice
Oranges	Papayas
Pineapples	Raisins
Satsumas	Tangerines
Watermelon	Dates, dried fruits

Low-Glycaemic Starches

The lowest-glycaemic starches that are the best starch choices include:

Amaranth	Bulgur
High-fibre multigrain bread	Low-carb bread
Millet	Quinoa
Pumpernickel	Sprouted bread
Whole-grain rye bread	Whole-grain wheat bread

Slightly higher-glycaemic starches that may be eaten on occasion, depending on how sensitive you are to them, include:

Brown rice	Corn tortillas
Melba toast	No-sugar-added, high-fibre cereals
Peas	Pita bread
Plain cooked oatmeal (not instant)	Spinach pasta

Starches you should avoid for the most part are:

Bagels	Bread (white flour)
Cakes	Cold cereals (except high-fibre)
Cookies	Crackers
Granola, granola bars	Muffins
Pretzels	Refined flours
Rice	Rice cakes
Semolina pasta	White sugar

GOOD FATS

Saturated fats typically come from animals (e.g. those found in fatty meats) as well as full-fat dairy products and tropical oils like palm oil and coconut oil. As a rule of thumb, they tend to be more solid at room temperature. When you have a lot of saturated fat in your diet, your liver responds by making more cholesterol, especially LDL (the bad cholesterol). This raises your blood cholesterol level. It is the most harmful type of fat you can eat. (However, see Chapter 2 for a discussion of why coconut oil may not act the same way as other saturated fats.)

Unsaturated fats (polyunsaturated and monounsaturated) have less of an effect on elevating blood cholesterol levels than saturated fats. Polyunsaturated fats come mainly from plants. They are liquid at room temperature. Eating polyunsaturated fat can reduce blood cholesterol levels.

Monounsaturated fats such as olive oil are mainly found in foods that come from plants. They are liquid at room temperature and can reduce blood cholesterol levels, but they're not as effective as polyunsaturated fats.

They can, however, raise HDL cholesterol (the good kind of cholesterol) levels.

Trans-fatty acids are produced when fats are hydrogenated. Hydrogenated fats like margarine and shortening are unsaturated fats that are made to be more solid at room temperature. Trans-fats can elevate LDL cholesterol levels.

The worst fats for your heart are saturated fats such as those found in fatty meats, full-fat dairy products and trans-fatty acids.

FATS

Saturated	Monounsaturated ('Good' Fat)	Polyunsaturated ('Good' Fat)	Hydrogenated/ Trans-Fats
Beef	Avocados	Almonds	Vegetable margarines
Lamb	Canola oil	Corn oil	Hydrogenated oil as
Pork	Cashews	Cottonseed oil	an ingredient in
Poultry	Olives	Filberts	processed foods
Milk/dairy	Olive oil	Fish	Partially hydrogenated
Brazil nuts	Peanuts	Flaxseeds	oil in processed
Butter	Peanut butter	Flaxseed oil	foods
Cheese	Peanut oil	Mayonnaise	
Chocolate		Pecans	
Coconut*		Safflower oil	
Coconut oil*		Sesame seeds	
Lard		Sesame oil	
Macadamia nuts		Soybean oil	
Palm oil		Sunflower oil	
Pistachios		Sunflower seeds	
		Walnuts	

*See Chapter 2 for information on coconut, coconut oil, and the potentially positive effects of medium-chain triglycerides.

Every meal or snack should have a serving of good fat. Some ways to add good fats into your diet are as follows:

- Toss a little bit of olive oil and a few sesame seeds on your salad.
- Add two to three small slices of avocado to a meal.
- Eat a handful of olives alongside a low-fat piece of protein and vegetables.
- Have a tablespoon of peanuts for a snack.
- Use olive oil when sautéing (versus butter – olive oil has 1.8 grams of saturated fat per tablespoon compared to 7 grams in butter).

TREATS

There are certain foods that should be considered treats and eaten in very limited quantities, if at all, when you are trying to lose weight or maintain weight loss. Here they are:

- fattier cuts of meat (e.g. prime rib), smoked meats (e.g. bacon)
- higher-glycaemic starches (e.g. plain white pasta, white bread)
- puddings (cake, biscuits, ice cream, sweets)
- alcohol
- sugared fizzy drinks

WHAT IS A SERVING SIZE?

I can almost guarantee you that the recommended serving size or portion of whatever food you are eating is probably smaller that you think it is! When I first started keeping track of serving sizes, I was amazed to find that my idea of a small lunchtime bowl of pasta was actually two to three servings. That plump chicken breast – two servings. And one of those really nice, big, fat-free blueberry muffins? Four servings of starch! The fundamental truth here: You will often overestimate the serving sizes of foods, but you'll rarely underestimate them.

You can walk around with food scales in your pocket – not particularly practical – or you can learn to eyeball fairly accurately a serving by comparing certain foods and serving sizes with common objects. Let's start with the definition of a meal-sized serving:

- Vegetables – one serving of vegetables is
    - 35g raw, chopped, or cooked
    - 200ml vegetable juice (try to stick with the low-sodium varieties, or juice it yourself)
    - 55g raw, leafy greens (like salad, spinach, etc.)
- Starch – one serving of starch is
    - 1 slice whole-wheat bread
    - half a whole-wheat bagel or muffin
    - 85g cooked whole-grain cereal, pasta, brown rice, cooked beans, corn, potatoes, rice or sweet potatoes
    - half a small potato or sweet potato, or 1 red potato
    - 2 slices melba toast, unseasoned
    - half a small corn tortilla
    - 100g popcorn
- Beef/pork/lamb – 85g
- Fish – 140g
- Poultry – 170g
- Cheese – 30g regular (55g low-fat)
- Egg – 2 eggs
- Fats – one serving of fat is
    - 1 tablespoon oil (i.e. olive, flaxseed, coconut)
    - 1 tablespoon low-fat mayonnaise (1 teaspoon regular mayonnaise)
    - 1 tablespoon oil and vinegar dressing
    - 5 large olives, 7 smaller olives
    - eighth of a medium-sized avocado
    - 1 teaspoon butter
    - 30g nuts without the shells, or 2 tablespoons peanut butter (snack-sized serving)
- Fruits – one serving of fruit is
    - 10 fresh cherries
    - 2 small tangerines or clementines
    - 140g berries
    - 1 small peach, apple or orange
    - 1 medium plum or nectarine
    - half a medium to large grapefruit or orange
    - 100g tinned fruit
    - 85g cut/cubed fruit (e.g. melon, papaya)

- 200ml juice
- 35g dried fruit
- Dairy products – one serving of dairy products is
  - 115ml low-fat milk
  - 115g fat-free or low-fat plain yogurt
  - 115g low-fat ricotta or cottage cheese

Not quite convinced that you're underestimating how much food you're eating? How much portions of popcorn do you think are in a medium-sized bag of popcorn? Would you be surprised to hear that it has eight full servings? Have you ever shared a bag of popcorn with eight people? More likely, you've eaten a whole bag yourself! (I have!)

How about that prime rib and baked potato dinner out? The typical amount of prime rib is 370 grams, or more than four servings of beef! And the large baked potato on the side? It's equivalent to four actual potato servings. Enough to feed a family of four!

What about those giant cinnamon buns that assault us at malls and airports? One is the equivalent of four starch servings! (Not to mention all the extra sugar!)

How to Eyeball Portions

Now that you're more familiar with the concept of a real portion size versus portions in our supersized food culture, let's talk about how to eyeball portions.

Amount	Is the size of ...
115g	A closed fist
85g	An ice cream scooper
2 tablespoons	A ping-pong ball
1 teaspoon	The top of your thumb from tip to joint
Meat, 85g	A deck of cards or a cassette tape
Cheese, 30g	Four stacked dice
Half a bagel	A hockey puck
1 medium-sized fruit	A tennis ball

Tips

Finally, here are two important tips to remember about portions:

- First, be careful when you're dealing with any pre-packaged foods that you assume are single serving, such as bottled juices, sweetened teas, a bag of crisps and so forth. Read the food label to see what the serving size is, then check to see the total size of the product. You may be looking at calories for a serving of juice or crisps, only to discover that the bottle or package you have is actually two servings.
- Second, whenever you can, measure out one serving and put it on a plate. Don't put the entire box, bowl, bag or platter on the table in front of you, or you will overestimate the serving amount. If a serving of cereal is 50 grams, take the time to weigh it, because until you are very good at eyeballing and are familiar with sizes, if you just shake the cereal into a bowl, you're likely to overestimate.

THE 'DESSERT' QUIZ

One of the main ways you can gauge how effectively you are eating is by taking this quiz. (Sorry, it has nothing to do with dessert, but it's a quiz for you to take instead of eating dessert!) Around 1 to 3 hours after eating, ask yourself:

- Was I hungry or dissatisfied soon after eating?
- Am I having any sweet cravings?
- Do I feel the need to snack before my next meal?
- Was I still feeling tired after I last ate?
- Is my thinking fuzzy?
- Am I feeling hyper, jittery, shaky, nervous or speedy?
- Is my pulse racing?
- Am I feeling sleepy or spaced out?
- Am I feeling depressed or sad?

The more 'yes' answers you have, the more likely it is that you did not eat the right foods for you. If you eat a meal that's right for you, you'll feel full, satisfied, energetic, free of cravings and won't be hungry again until it's time to eat your next meal.

If you are keeping a weight-loss journal, keeping track of how you feel after each meal will help you to identify those meals that work the best for you, and will also help you identify food sensitivities, food allergies, eating triggers and foods that derail your weight-loss efforts.

YOUR OWN PERSONAL FOOD HIT LIST

In the end, no food is off-limits. But you will have to come up with your own personal 'hit list' of foods to limit or avoid. These would include:

- Foods to which you are allergic
- Foods to which you are sensitive
- Foods that give you diarrhoea, stomach cramps or abdominal pain
- Foods and drinks that cause you to feel shaky or sweaty
- Foods that make your pulse go up
- Foods that make you hungrier than ever
- Foods where you just can't eat one, so you eat the whole box, bag or carton
- Foods that always seem to bloat you up for a few days
- Foods that make your skin break out
- Foods that make you totally exhausted.

A weight-loss journal/food diary or tracking system, along with daily weigh-ins (if you can stand it), can really be a help. You'll see patterns after a few weeks of tracking that start to reveal some of the unique aspects of your own physiology and way of eating and responding to foods and exercise.

I can't tell you which foods will be on your personal list, because that list will be unique to you. Some people can drink a cup or two of coffee; other people find that it makes them shaky and messes up their blood sugar for the day. Some people can use dairy products, whereas others find that dairy gives them a stomach-ache, bloats them up for a day or two and stalls weight loss. In my own case, here are a few examples:

- I'm allergic to tree fruits (apples, pears, peaches, plums, cherries) and tree nuts (walnuts, pecans, etc.).
- I cannot eat just one piece of chocolate, so I don't eat any.
- Drinking fruit juice (like orange juice) makes me incredibly hungry.
- If I use a lot of soy sauce, I carry an extra pound or two of water weight for a few days. If I use the low-sodium type, it's much less of a problem.

So it's going to be up to you to determine which foods maximize your metabolism, help you to feel your best and help you to lose weight most effectively while not feeling hungry, bloated, constipated and so on.

EGG AND PANCAKE RECIPES

Omelet

Servings: 1   *Degree of Difficulty: Easy*
Preparation Time: 15 minutes   *Time from Start to Eating: 15 minutes*

Amount	Ingredients	Preparation
1	Omega-3 egg	
2	Egg whites	(55–85g egg whites)
2 tablespoons	Water	
	Cooking spray	

OPTIONS: Filling Ingredients

4 leaves	Fresh spinach	Raw (washed)
25g	Mushrooms	Diced
45g	Tomatoes	Diced
50g	Turkey, lean	Cooked, diced
2 tablespoons	Onions	Diced
25g	Peppers	Diced
25g	Broccoli	Steamed, chopped

In a small bowl or measuring cup, combine omega-3 egg, egg whites and water. Beat until thoroughly combined.

Heat pan over medium-high heat. Remove pan from heat, spray with cooking spray, wait a few seconds and then return to heat. Pour in egg mixture. Almost immediately, drag a rubber spatula through the mixture in one direction, pulling the cooked thin layer towards you. (If you're adding optional filling ingredients, add them now.)

With rubber spatula, go around entire edge of omelet in pan, lifting and making sure the omelet isn't sticking anywhere. (If you shake the pan, the omelet should slide.) When the omelet is done to your liking (2–3 minutes should be fine), gently slide it onto a plate, folding in half. If you like really well-done, dry omelets, you can turn the omelet over after 2 minutes so that both sides are exposed directly to the heat in the bottom of the pan.

Recipe Nutritional Breakdown	Amount per Serving
Calories	125
Fat (g)	5
Saturated (g)	1.5
Polyunsaturated (g)	1
Monounsaturated (g)	3
Cholesterol (mg)	180
Carbohydrates (g)	7
Fibre (g)	0
Sugars (g)	0
Protein (g)	13

COMPLETE MEAL SUGGESTION

Omelet with a spinach, tomato and mushroom filling served with a slice of whole-wheat toast.

Meal Nutritional Breakdown	Amount per Serving
Calories	213
Fat (g)	6
Saturated (g)	2
Polyunsaturated (g)	2
Monounsaturated (g)	3
Cholesterol (mg)	180
Carbohydrates (g)	24
Fibre (g)	2.5
Sugars (g)	0
Protein (g)	17

Buckwheat Pancakes

Servings: 3
Preparation Time: 5 minutes

Degree of Difficulty: Moderate
Time from Start to Eating: 20 minutes

Amount	Ingredients	Preparation
225ml	Low-fat buttermilk or fromage frais	
1	Omega-3 egg	Separate whites from yolk
2 tablespoons	Corn oil	
6 tablespoons	Buckwheat flour	
6 tablespoons	All-purpose flour	
½ teaspoon	Sugar	
¼ teaspoon	Salt	
1 teaspoon	Baking soda	
5	Dried apricots	Chopped
4 tablespoons	Pecans	Toasted and chopped
	Cooking spray	

In a mixing bowl, combine buttermilk, egg yolk and corn oil. In a copper bowl (if you don't have a copper bowl, any clean cold bowl will do), whip egg whites to soft peaks. (Separating and whipping egg whites results in lighter pancakes.)

In another bowl, mix together both flours, sugar, salt and baking soda. Add apricots and pecans to flour mixture. Combine dry ingredients with buttermilk mixture. Fold egg whites into mixture.

Heat a griddle or large frying pan to medium-hot. Remove pan from heat, spray with cooking spray, wait a few seconds and then return to heat. Ladle batter to form 4-inch pancakes. Once bubbles form on the top of pancakes, flip them over and cook them on the other side for about 2–3 minutes. Continue until all batter has been made into pancakes.

Recipe Nutritional Breakdown	Amount per Serving
Calories	320
Fat (g)	16
Saturated (g)	2
Polyunsaturated (g)	4
Monounsaturated (g)	9
Cholesterol (mg)	63
Carbohydrates (g)	38
Fibre (g)	3.5
Sugars (g)	4
Protein (g)	10

COMPLETE MEAL SUGGESTION

Top pancakes with sliced peaches, sliced strawberries and serve with 85g cooked turkey breast slices.

Meal Nutritional Breakdown	Amount per Serving
Calories	514
Fat (g)	19
Saturated (g)	3
Polyunsaturated (g)	5
Monounsaturated (g)	9
Cholesterol (mg)	122
Carbohydrates (g)	53
Fibre (g)	7
Sugars (g)	4
Protein (g)	36

Eggs Sardu

Servings: 6
Preparation Time: 20 minutes

Degree of Difficulty: Moderate
Time from Start to Eating: 20 minutes

This is a great brunch menu idea, and most of the preparation can be done in advance.

Amount	Ingredients	Preparation
1 teaspoon	Vinegar	
1 dozen	Omega-3 eggs	
6	Muffins or crumpets	If using muffins, split
115g	Yogurt cheese	
1 tablespoon	Lemon juice (fresh)	
1 pinch	Cayenne pepper	
1 teaspoon	Herbs de Provence	(Thyme, parsley, lavender, rosemary, basil, fennel, savoury, tarragon or similar mixture)
1 teaspoon	Salt	
	Pepper, to taste	
1 package	Chopped spinach, frozen	Defrosted and drained (285g package)
2	Tomatoes	Sliced, ¼-inch thick
1 tin	Artichoke hearts in water*	Rinsed and drained (395g tin)

*Do not use marinated artichokes.

Preheat oven to 400°F/200°C/GM6. In a large, wide pot, bring 2 pints of water to boil. Add vinegar to the water.

In a large bowl, crack eggs open (whole, do not beat or break), being careful not to leave any shell. (I crack each one in a small bowl, then add them into the big bowl to avoid problems.) Once water is boiling, reduce heat. Add eggs and adjust heat so that water simmers. If you have an instant-read thermometer (and you should!), the temperature should be about 180°F/80°C.

While eggs are cooking, rinse egg bowl and fill it with water and ice cubes. After eggs have been poaching for 3 minutes, remove them using a slotted spoon and place them in the ice bath. This will stop the cooking process immediately. The cooking water should be kept on the hob, covered and hot.

Place open muffins or crumpets on a dry baking sheet and set aside.

In a small bowl, combine yogurt cheese, lemon juice, cayenne, herbs de Provence, salt and pepper. Microwave for 30 seconds on 70 per cent power.

Combine spinach with yogurt sauce. Taste. Adjust seasonings to your liking.

Place the muffins/crumpets on baking sheet in oven to toast. This will take about 3 minutes, but keep an eye on them.

Place two muffin halves/crumpets on each plate. Top with tomato slice and artichoke heart.

When all plates are ready, take two eggs from ice bath and return them to hot water for about 30 seconds. Remove them with slotted spoon and place on muffins, directly on top of the artichoke hearts. Now place some of the spinach and yogurt mix on the side and serve.

Recipe Nutritional Breakdown	Amount per Serving
Calories	369
Fat (g)	12
Saturated (g)	4
Polyunsaturated (g)	3
Monounsaturated (g)	6
Cholesterol (mg)	362
Carbohydrates (g)	47
Fibre (g)	4
Sugars (g)	0
Protein (g)	21

COMPLETE MEAL SUGGESTION

Serve with a side of sliced apples and orange sections.

Meal Nutritional Breakdown	Amount per Serving
Calories	441
Fat (g)	12
Saturated (g)	4
Polyunsaturated (g)	3
Monounsaturated (g)	6
Cholesterol (mg)	362
Carbohydrates (g)	66
Fibre (g)	7.5
Sugars (g)	0
Protein (g)	21

Huevos Rancheros

Servings: 1

Preparation Time: 20 minutes

Degree of Difficulty: Easy

Time from Start to Eating: 20 minutes

Amount	Ingredients	Preparation
2	Corn tortillas	Heated in microwave
50g	Black beans and rice*	Heated in microwave
2	Omega-3 eggs	
1 tablespoon	Salsa	
3 tablespoons	Bell peppers (red, green)	Chopped
2 slices	Avocado	(⅛ of an avocado)
Sprigs	Cilantro	Optional
	Cooking spray	

*I make this dish when I have beans and rice left over. If you're craving Mexican but don't have the leftovers, you can use black beans (tinned) without the rice, or you can use Uncle Ben's converted rice and cook it in advance of breakfast (it only adds about 20 minutes to your time and there isn't much preparation). Uncle Ben's converted rice has a lower glycaemic index than other white rice.

Heat tortillas and beans/rice separately in microwave. (Sprinkle a few drops of water on tortillas before heating.) Remove from microwave and keep warm until ready to plate. (Tortillas will dry out quickly, so leave them covered.)

Heat pan over medium-high heat. Remove pan from heat, spray with cooking spray, wait a few seconds and then return to heat. Crack both eggs into a bowl. Pour the whole eggs into the hot pan. Cook to your preference (over easy or sunny-side-up are traditional).

While eggs are cooking, place tortillas on plates, then add beans and rice on top in a thin layer (I spread them all over). Add cooked eggs and top with salsa, bell peppers and avocado. Garnish with cilantro sprigs if desired.

Recipe Nutritional Breakdown	Amount per Serving
Calories	367
Fat (g)	15
Saturated (g)	4
Polyunsaturated (g)	4
Monounsaturated (g)	9
Cholesterol (mg)	360
Carbohydrates (g)	42
Fibre (g)	6
Sugars (g)	0
Protein (g)	17

COMPLETE MEAL SUGGESTION

Serve with apple and orange slices (half of a whole apple and half of a whole orange).

Meal Nutritional Breakdown	Amount per Serving
Calories	441
Fat (g)	16
Saturated (g)	4
Polyunsaturated (g)	4
Monounsaturated (g)	9
Cholesterol (mg)	360
Carbohydrates (g)	62
Fibre (g)	9
Sugars (g)	0
Protein (g)	18

SAUCES AND DRESSINGS

Buttermilk Ranch Dressing

Servings: 20 (1 tablespoon/serving)   *Degree of Difficulty: Moderate*
Preparation Time: 5 minutes   *Time from Start to Eating: 1–3 hours*

Amount	Ingredients	Preparation
55g	Onion	Chopped fine
1 tablespoon	Cider vinegar	(Any vinegar is okay)
1 tablespoon	Olive oil	
1 tablespoon	Mustard	Dijon, brown, whatever mustard you enjoy
2 tablespoons	Parsley	Chopped
2 tablespoons	Chives	Chopped
1 teaspoon	Salt	
	Pepper to taste	
55g	Yogurt, low-fat	(Use yogurt cheese if you prefer a thicker dressing)
170g	Low-fat buttermilk or fromage frais	

Combine onion, vinegar, oil, mustard, parsley, chives, salt and pepper in bowl of food processor or blender. Process or blend for a minute or two, until well combined. Combine yogurt and buttermilk in small bowl, then add oil–vinegar mixture to it and stir. Cover with plastic wrap and refrigerate at least 1 hour before using. Flavours develop best with several hours of refrigeration.

Recipe Nutritional Breakdown	Amount per Serving
Calories	16
Fat (g)	1
Saturated (g)	0
Polyunsaturated (g)	0
Monounsaturated (g)	1
Cholesterol (mg)	1
Carbohydrates (g)	1
Fibre (g)	0
Sugars (g)	1
Protein (g)	1

Roasted Garlic Sauce

Servings: 4   *Degree of Difficulty: Easy*
Preparation Time: 5 minutes   *Time from Start to Eating: 1 hour*

Amount	Ingredients	Preparation
4	Garlic heads*	About 30 cloves, separated and peeled
1 teaspoon	Olive oil	
115g	Yogurt cheese	
	Salt, to taste	
	Pepper, to taste	

* You can purchase already peeled garlic cloves at most grocery stores.

Preheat oven to 375°F/190°C/GM5. On large piece of aluminium foil, place garlic cloves and drizzle with olive oil. Fold up corners of foil to make a closed, sealed packet, then place in oven over baking sheet. Leave in oven for about an hour. You'll know the garlic is done when you smell a wonderful aroma coming from the oven and garlic cloves will look slightly toasted.

Remove garlic packet from oven, allowing cloves to cool slightly. Add them to the bowl of a food processor and add yogurt cheese. Process until well combined. Adjust seasoning with salt and pepper.

Recipe Nutritional Breakdown	Amount per Serving
Calories	50
Fat (g)	2
Saturated (g)	1
Polyunsaturated (g)	0
Monounsaturated (g)	1
Cholesterol (mg)	3
Carbohydrates (g)	5
Fibre (g)	0
Sugars (g)	0
Protein (g)	3

Ginger Soy Vinaigrette

Amount	Ingredients	Preparation
3 tablespoons	Sesame oil	
3 tablespoons	Corn oil	
1 tablespoon	Tamari sauce	(naturally brewed soy sauce)
3 tablespoons	Ginger	Thinly sliced
3 tablespoons	Mayonnaise	Low-fat
1 tablespoon	Mirin	(Japanese sweet wine, rice wine)
pinch	Cayenne pepper	

Combine ingredients in blender and blend until all ingredients are well combined and ginger is minced. Adjust flavours to taste. Refrigerate until ready to use.

Recipe Nutritional Breakdown	Amount per Serving
Calories	29
Fat (g)	3
Saturated (g)	0
Polyunsaturated (g)	1
Monounsaturated (g)	1
Cholesterol (mg)	1
Carbohydrates (g)	0
Fibre (g)	0
Sugars (g)	0
Protein (g)	2

Pesto

Servings: 8
Preparation Time: 5 minutes

Degree of Difficulty: Easy
Time from Start to Eating: 5 minutes

Amount	Ingredients	Preparation
60g	Basil leaves	Fresh, rinsed and dried
2 tablespoons	Pine nuts	(Or walnuts, if preferred)
2	Garlic cloves	Peeled and chopped
115ml	Olive oil	
2 tablespoons	Parmesan cheese	Freshly grated
1 tablespoon	Romano cheese	Freshly grated
	Salt	

Put basil, nuts, garlic cloves and olive oil in blender or food processor. Blend on high until well combined (should be mushy), scraping down sides if necessary. Add freshly grated cheeses to mixture and pulse again until well combined. Add salt.

Use pesto as a spread on bread, or as a sauce on pasta or meat. It's the taste of summer!

The nutritional breakdown might scare you, but remember this replaces butter or fat. It's lower in saturated fat and tastes amazing.

Recipe Nutritional Breakdown	Amount per Serving
Calories	161
Fat (g)	17
Saturated (g)	3
Polyunsaturated (g)	2
Monounsaturated (g)	11
Cholesterol (mg)	4
Carbohydrates (g)	1
Fibre (g)	0.5
Sugars (g)	0
Protein (g)	2

Sun-Dried Tomato Topping

Servings: 4   *Degree of Difficulty: Easy*

Preparation Time: 5 minutes   *Time from Start to Eating: 30 minutes*

Amount	Ingredients	Preparation
170g	Sun-dried tomatoes	Dry, not in oil
225g	Yogurt cheese	
1 tablespoon	Garlic	Minced
	Salt, to taste	
	Pepper, to taste	

Reconstitute sun-dried tomatoes according to package directions. (This usually means putting in a bowl, covering with boiled water and setting aside for 20 minutes or so, until tender.) Drain and pat dry.

In the bowl of a food processor, combine sun-dried tomatoes with yogurt cheese and garlic. Process until smooth. Adjust seasoning with salt and pepper.

This is excellent on poached chicken!

Recipe Nutritional Breakdown	Amount per Serving
Calories	72
Fat (g)	1
Saturated (g)	0.5
Polyunsaturated (g)	0
Monounsaturated (g)	0
Cholesterol (mg)	3
Carbohydrates (g)	12
Fibre (g)	2
Sugars (g)	0
Protein (g)	5

CHICKEN

Brined Chicken Breast

Degree of Difficulty: Easy

Preparation Time: Overnight

Time from Start to Eating: Not applicable

Amount	Ingredients	Preparation
50g	Salt	
65g	Sugar	
Herbs/seasonings	Your preference	
900g	Chicken breast (skin, bones optional)	

Brining is a method of preparing a chicken before cooking. Why brine? Chicken breasts tend to dry out easily if overcooked. Brining helps keep the chicken moist and adds flavour to the meat. Think of it as a moisturizing marinade.

To make brine mixture, boil 425ml water. Put salt, sugar and seasonings in a large bowl. Pour boiled water into bowl and stir to dissolve salt and sugar. Once dissolved, add ice cubes to cool down, then add 425ml cold water.

Pour brining mixture into a sealable container. Add chicken breasts and make sure they are covered by brine. Put container in refrigerator.

Alternative: Put in extra-large sized bags that have a zip lock, making sure to get all the air out of the bag.

Don't brine longer than 24 hours, or chicken can become rubbery.

Now use the chicken in any of your recipes, cooking as indicated. (But be sure to rinse and pat dry brined chicken before cooking.)

Note: If you brine meat, you do *not* need to salt the meat again before cooking.

Poached Chicken Breast

Servings: 4 115-gram servings   *Degree of Difficulty: Easy*
Preparation Time: 20 minutes   *Time from Start to Eating: 30 minutes*

Amount	Ingredient	Preparation
455g	Chicken breast	Bones and skin removed

Using a covered pan, fill two-thirds full of water. Bring to a boil, then reduce to a simmer. (I prefer to use brined chicken breast, but it's not necessary.) Add chicken breast, which will drop temperature of water. Keep heat on and use instant-read thermometer. Temperature should come back up to 190°F/85°C, not to a boil. (Boiling makes the chicken rubbery.) Once water is to temperature, cover, reduce heat and leave for about 15 minutes, checking occasionally that it's not too hot or cool.

Cook chicken breast until internal temperature reads 160°F/70°C, meaning chicken has been cooked through. (It'll continue cooking a few minutes after removed from water, to reach an internal temperature of 165°F/75°C.) Remove chicken from water, put on cutting board and cover with foil, letting sit for 5 to 10 minutes. (This is called 'resting the meat'. You never want to cut meat that is straight from the oven or heat source – the juices will all run out and the meat will be dry.)

You now have a great building block for many low-fat meals and snacks.

Recipe Nutritional Breakdown	Amount per Serving
Calories	170
Fat (g)	3
Saturated (g)	1
Polyunsaturated (g)	1
Monounsaturated (g)	1
Cholesterol (mg)	87
Carbohydrates (g)	0
Fibre (g)	0
Sugars (g)	0
Protein (g)	33

Chicken with Mushroom Sauce

Servings: 4
Preparation Time: 25 minutes

Degree of Difficulty: Moderate
Time from Start to Eating: 45 minutes

Amount	Ingredients	Preparation
455g	Brined Chicken Breast	(page 195)
1 tablespoon	Peanut oil	(Or olive oil or corn oil)
170g	Mushrooms	Quartered
1 tablespoon	Tomato paste	
1 tablespoon	Brandy	Optional
225ml	White wine*	heated in microwave
425ml	Chicken broth	Fat-free, low-sodium –
		heated in microwave
1 tablespoon	Cornstarch	
	Cooking spray	

* Good enough quality to drink with meal. Chardonnay and chenin blanc are good choices.

* Throughout the recipes, you'll see the specification to warm a liquid in the microwave before you add it to a recipe. This is a chef's trick to help keep your cooking time as short as possible. If you heat liquids, then they are warmer when you add them in with other ingredients and the dish will come to a boil far more quickly, making for quicker preparation and less time in the kitchen!

Preheat oven to 400°F/200°C/GM6. Remove chicken from brine, rinse, then dry with paper towels.

Heat large frying pan over medium-high heat. Remove pan from heat, spray with cooking spray, wait a few seconds and then return to the heat. Add chicken breasts and place heavy pan or weight on top of chicken so that browning is enhanced. After 4 or 5 minutes, turn chicken over, again adding weight. Once both sides are browned, remove chicken from pan, place on sprayed baking sheet and put in oven for 25 minutes or so (until done).

In hot frying pan, add oil. Once oil is very hot, add mushrooms. Shake pan a bit, but do not stir. After 5 minutes or so, stir mushrooms around. Cook them over medium-high heat until well browned and there is no visible moisture left in pan.

Remove pan from hob and add brandy. Return pan back to hob, tilting pan slightly. The brandy should ignite. This is a flambé. If you use an electric cooker, you need to use a long (fireplace) match to ignite brandy. Once lit, shake pan gently until blue flames go out. (This is a really fun, impressive cooking technique. If it scares you, skip it. Don't add the brandy. Just go to next step.)

Add tomato paste to pan and stir with mushrooms. Add white wine, stir well and scrape bottom of pan to get up all the tomato paste and browned bits from the chicken and mushrooms. (Adds great flavour to the sauce!) Cook over medium-high heat until wine is almost gone; liquid in bottom of pan should be slightly syrupy. Now add chicken broth. Let this cook for as long as it takes for chicken to finish.

Once chicken is done, remove from oven and let sit on cutting board for at least 5 minutes. This is called resting the meat. It's important for flavour, so don't rush this.

While chicken is resting, mix cornstarch and 60ml cold water in small cup or bowl. Pour this into mushroom sauce to slightly thicken it. Stir well to combine. Mixture should not be as thick as gravy – it's a beautiful glossy sauce that will impress all your guests (or family, though they are harder to impress ...).

Cut chicken breasts in half, portion onto plates and top with mushrooms and sauce.

Recipe Nutritional Breakdown	Amount per Serving
Calories	303
Fat (g)	8
Saturated (g)	2
Polyunsaturated (g)	2
Monounsaturated (g)	3
Cholesterol (mg)	96
Carbohydrates (g)	6
Fibre (g)	1
Sugars (g)	0
Protein (g)	39

COMPLETE MEAL SUGGESTION

Serve with 85g steamed broccoli with fresh lemon juice.

Meal Nutritional Breakdown	Amount per Serving
Calories	331
Fat (g)	9
Saturated (g)	2
Polyunsaturated (g)	2
Monounsaturated (g)	3
Cholesterol (mg)	96
Carbohydrates (g)	12
Fibre (g)	1
Sugars (g)	0
Protein (g)	41

Chicken Salad

Servings: 4

Preparation Time: 5 minutes

Degree of Difficulty: Easy

Time from Start to Eating: 1 hour

Amount	Ingredients	Preparation
455g	Poached Chicken Breast	Cut into bite-sized pieces
1	Celery stalk	Diced
55g	Yogurt cheese	
1 tablespoon	Dijon mustard	
1 tablespoon	Tarragon	Diced
	Salt, to taste	
	Pepper, to taste	

In a bowl, combine chicken and celery. In another bowl, combine yogurt cheese, mustard and tarragon. Add salt and pepper to yogurt cheese mixture. (If it is too tangy, you can combine a tablespoon of low-fat mayonnaise or low-fat soured cream with yogurt cheese.) Once it's to your liking, add small amounts of sauce to chicken and celery, just enough to combine.

You can eat this straight away, but tarragon flavour develops better if left for an hour.

Recipe Nutritional Breakdown	Amount per Serving
Calories	184
Fat (g)	4
Saturated (g)	1
Polyunsaturated (g)	1
Monounsaturated (g)	1
Cholesterol (mg)	88
Carbohydrates (g)	2
Fibre (g)	0
Sugars (g)	0
Protein (g)	34

COMPLETE MEAL SUGGESTION

Serve with 2 rye crackers and 1 cut-up apple.

Meal Nutritional Breakdown	Amount per Serving
Calories	349
Fat (g)	5
Saturated (g)	1
Polyunsaturated (g)	1
Monounsaturated (g)	1
Cholesterol (mg)	88
Carbohydrates (g)	41
Fibre (g)	7
Sugars (g)	0
Protein (g)	36

Roasted Garlic Chicken

Servings: 4 *Degree of Difficulty: Easy*
Preparation Time: 10 minutes *Time from Start to Eating: 90 minutes*

Amount	Ingredients	Preparation
225ml	Roasted Garlic Sauce	(page 191)
455g	Poached Chicken Breast	(page 196)

Spoon roasted garlic topping on poached chicken, then place chicken on baking sheet under the grill for 3 or 4 minutes until topping is browned.

Recipe Nutritional Breakdown	Amount per Serving
Calories	220
Fat (g)	5
Saturated (g)	2
Polyunsaturated (g)	0
Monounsaturated (g)	2
Cholesterol (mg)	91
Carbohydrates (g)	5
Fibre (g)	0
Sugars (g)	0
Protein (g)	36

COMPLETE MEAL SUGGESTION

Serve with 85g sautéed mushrooms and 105g baked yam (baked while roasting garlic) per serving.

Meal Nutritional Breakdown	Amount per Serving
Calories	347
Fat (g)	6
Saturated (g)	2
Polyunsaturated (g)	1
Monounsaturated (g)	2
Cholesterol (mg)	90
Carbohydrates (g)	35
Fibre (g)	5
Sugars (g)	0
Protein (g)	38

Pasta Salad with Chicken or Turkey

Servings: 6
Preparation Time: 20 minutes

Degree of Difficulty: Easy
Time from Start to Eating: 20 minutes

Amount	Ingredients	Preparation
680g	Spinach pasta	Boiled, al dente, rinsed with cold water
2 tablespoons	Pesto	(page 193)
340g	Turkey breast or Poached Chicken Breast	Skinless, cubed
170–225g	Tomatoes	Sliced (I prefer cherry tomatoes for this)
115g	Artichoke hearts	Tinned, rinsed, quartered
170g	Broccoli	Steamed, chopped (use stems too)
2 tablespoons	Lemon juice	(juice from half a lemon, no seeds)
	Salt, to taste	
	Pepper, to taste	
115g	Part-skim milk mozzarella	Bite-sized pieces, room temperature

Combine all ingredients in large bowl except mozzarella and toss thoroughly. Place in separate bowls and top with mozzarella. If you want a more elegant presentation, add basil leaves and lemon zest.

Note: If you plunge vegetables into an ice bath directly from boiling water, you stop the cooking immediately and generally keep the vegetables a bright green colour.

Recipe Nutritional Breakdown	Amount per Serving
Calories	339
Fat (g)	10
Saturated (g)	3
Polyunsaturated (g)	1
Monounsaturated (g)	4
Cholesterol (mg)	50
Carbohydrates (g)	33
Fibre (g)	3.5
Sugars (g)	0
Protein (g)	29

COMPLETE MEAL SUGGESTION

I really like this recipe because it's a great leftover! I zap it in the microwave for 45 seconds on 70 per cent power and it's amazing. I think this is a great summer meal when served with some fresh corn on the cob (I microwave under fresh vegetable setting). I don't butter my corn. I usually just add some pepper and, if I'm really feeling decadent, then I rub a bit of pesto on it. For dessert, I think a fresh, really ripe peach is ideal! Nectarines and other summer fruits are all fine.

Meal Nutritional Breakdown	Amount per Serving
Calories	466
Fat (g)	11
Saturated (g)	4
Polyunsaturated (g)	2
Monounsaturated (g)	5
Cholesterol (mg)	50
Carbohydrates (g)	63
Fibre (g)	8
Sugars (g)	0
Protein (g)	33

PORK

Pulled Pork

Servings: 12
Preparation Time: 20 minutes

Degree of Difficulty: Moderate
Time from Start to Eating: 7 hours

Amount	Ingredients	Preparation
1	Onion	Chopped
3	Carrots	Chopped
3	Celery stalks	Chopped
3	Garlic cloves	Peeled and chopped
2 tablespoons	Cumin, ground	
1 tablespoon	Coriander seed, ground	
1 teaspoon	Cayenne pepper	
1.35 kilos	Pork loin	
225ml	Red wine*	
795g	Tomatoes	Chopped (tinned are fine)
900g	Chicken broth	Fat-free, low-sodium
1	Bay leaf	
	Salt, to taste	
	Pepper, to taste	
	Cooking spray	

*Use a wine that is of quality to drink; cabernet sauvignon or a hearty burgundy is great.

Heat a heavy frying pan over medium heat. Remove pan from heat, spray with cooking spray, wait a few seconds and then return to heat. Add onion, carrots and celery to frying pan and stir. Reduce heat if too high – you want to sweat the onions, not brown them. Cook for 10 minutes, stirring occasionally.

Add garlic, cumin, coriander and cayenne pepper. Stir well, cooking for 1 minute. Remove ingredients from pan, placing directly into slow cooker.

Return pan to hob over medium-high heat and respray with cooking spray. Add pork loin to brown (if too long, cut it in half and brown in two batches). Do not turn pork for 3 minutes or so. Once there is good colour on it, turn and continue browning. Do this until it is fully browned. Add loin to slow cooker.

Add wine and deglaze pan. (This means keep heat on and stir constantly, scraping up all bits on bottom of pan. This stuff adds great flavour to the sauce!) Continue cooking until wine is reduced by half. Add liquid to slow cooker.

Add tinned tomatoes, chicken broth and bay leaf to slow cooker. Cover and set slow cooker to high.

Let pork cook all day or overnight. After it has cooked for at least 6 hours, remove cover and turn off cooker. Remove pork from sauce and put it on a cutting board to rest.

If sauce is too thin for you, further reduce by putting it in a pan over medium heat, cooking until reduced to your liking. This intensifies the flavour.

Strain sauce through a hand strainer or cheesecloth. Taste sauce and adjust seasonings with salt and pepper.

Once loin has rested (10 minutes or so should be fine), take two forks and start pulling pork in opposite directions to shred. I add the meat back to a container and pour the sauce directly over it.

This is great for leftovers and also for freezing!

Recipe Nutritional Breakdown	Amount per Serving
Calories	302
Fat (g)	12
Saturated (g)	4
Polyunsaturated (g)	1
Monounsaturated (g)	5
Cholesterol (mg)	94
Carbohydrates (g)	9
Fibre (g)	3
Sugars (g)	0
Protein (g)	36

COMPLETE MEAL SUGGESTION

Serve with 100g cooked pearl barley and 115g cooked spinach with fresh
lemon juice per serving.

Meal Nutritional Breakdown	Amount per Serving
Calories	421
Fat (g)	13
Saturated (g)	4
Polyunsaturated (g)	1
Monounsaturated (g)	5
Cholesterol (mg)	94
Carbohydrates (g)	34
Fibre (g)	8
Sugars (g)	0
Protein (g)	40

Pork Enchilada Casserole (Con Salsa Verde)

Servings: 6
Preparation Time: 25 minutes

Degree of Difficulty: Moderate
Time from Start to Eating: 1 hour

Amount	Ingredients	Preparation
455g	Tomatillos	Husked and rinsed, cut in half (Tomatillos are available in the produce section of many groceries, as well as Mexican and Latin American foods speciality sections or markets. You can also use tinned tomatillos.)
2 tablespoons	Sherry vinegar	
2 tins	Green chillies	Drained (115g tins)
2	Jalapeños	Chopped (remove ribs and seeds)
30g	Cilantro	Chopped
4	Garlic cloves	Peeled and chopped
1 tablespoon	Corn oil	
425ml	Chicken broth	Fat-free, low-sodium
	Salt, to taste	
	Pepper, to taste	
8	Corn tortillas	Cut in half for easier layering
675g	Pulled Pork	(page 205)
1 package	Peppers, red, green, yellow	Available ready to use in (450g bag)
115g	Monterey Jack or Cheddar cheese	Low-fat, grated

Turn on the grill. Place tomatillos and peppers on baking sheet and grill to brown, about 3 minutes. Remove and allow to cool slightly. Place tomatillos in bowl of food processor. Pour vinegar over baking sheet and scrape up brown bits from it. Pour this into food processor.

Set oven to 325°F/170°C/GM3.

Add chillies, jalapeños, cilantro, garlic, corn oil and chicken broth to food processor. Pulse until well combined. Adjust seasonings with salt and pepper.

In casserole dish, pour some of the tomatillo sauce on bottom to wet. Cover bottom with one layer of corn tortillas. Top with pulled pork and tomatillo sauce. Repeat layering until done. Top with cheese.

Bake in oven, uncovered, for 30 minutes or so.

Recipe Nutritional Breakdown	Amount per Serving
Calories	255
Fat (g)	9
Saturated (g)	3
Polyunsaturated (g)	3
Monounsaturated (g)	3
Cholesterol (mg)	37
Carbohydrates (g)	22
Fibre (g)	3
Sugars (g)	0
Protein (g)	22

COMPLETE MEAL SUGGESTION

Serve with a green salad that has apples, orange segments or pumpkin seeds on it with a simple vinaigrette.

Meal Nutritional Breakdown	Amount per Serving
Calories	479
Fat (g)	17
Saturated (g)	4
Polyunsaturated (g)	7
Monounsaturated (g)	5
Cholesterol (mg)	37
Carbohydrates (g)	62
Fibre (g)	11
Sugars (g)	0
Protein (g)	25

RED MEAT

Chili Con Carne with Beans

Servings: 8   *Degree of Difficulty: Easy*
Preparation Time: 20 minutes   *Time from Start to Eating: 30–45 minutes*

Amount	Ingredients	Preparation
2 tablespoons	Olive oil	
455–570g	Beef or bison, minced	
	Salt, to taste	
	Pepper, to taste	
1 tablespoon	Cumin	
1 tablespoon	Coriander, ground	
3 tablespoons	Chilli powder	
2 tablespoons	Tomato paste	
1	Onion	Diced
225g	Red and green peppers	Diced
2 tins	Kidney beans	Rinsed and drained (440g tins)
1 tin	Tomatoes, chopped	Low-sodium (795g tin)
2	Jalapeños	Seeded
	Cooking spray	

Heat large frying pan over medium-high heat. When pan is hot, remove from heat, spray with cooking spray and then return to heat. Add 1 table-spoon olive oil. When oil is hot, add beef, salt and pepper and stir, brown-ing meat. Add cumin, coriander, chilli powder and tomato paste. Cook for 2 more minutes, stirring well.

Put meat from pan in a bowl and set aside. Add remaining tablespoon of olive oil to pan. Add onions and peppers, stirring occasionally. Cook 10–15 minutes to develop flavour. Return meat to pan, stir well, then add kidney beans, tomatoes and jalapeños.

Cover and allow to simmer for approximately 20 minutes. Check seasonings. If you prefer spicier, in a small heavy frying pan over medium-high heat, add 1 tablespoon olive oil, then add more cumin, coriander, chilli powder and some cayenne pepper. Stir well, not allowing spices to burn. Add some chilli mixture from large pan to small pan, allowing spices to get incorporated into chilli. Return this mixture to chilli batch. Stir well, allow to simmer for 5 more minutes, then taste again.

Recipe Nutritional Breakdown	Amount per Serving
Calories	230
Fat (g)	8
Saturated (g)	2
Polyunsaturated (g)	1
Monounsaturated (g)	4
Cholesterol (mg)	49
Carbohydrates (g)	18
Fibre (g)	4
Sugars (g)	0
Protein (g)	23

COMPLETE MEAL SUGGESTION

Serve a bowl of chilli with a green salad with buttermilk ranch dressing, several baby carrots and a baked apple.

Meal Nutritional Breakdown	Amount per Serving
Calories	382
Fat (g)	9
Saturated (g)	2
Polyunsaturated (g)	1
Monounsaturated (g)	5
Cholesterol (mg)	50
Carbohydrates (g)	52
Fibre (g)	7
Sugars (g)	1
Protein (g)	27

Meatloaf

Servings: 6　　　　　　　　　　　　　　*Degree of Difficulty: Moderate*
Preparation Time: 30 minutes　　　　　*Time from Start to Eating: 90 minutes*

Amount	Ingredients	Preparation
1 teaspoon	Olive or vegetable oil	
115g	Onion	Chopped
70g	Carrot	Chopped
55g	Celery	Chopped
2	Garlic cloves	Minced
1 teaspoon	Cayenne pepper	
½ teaspoon	Thyme	
15g	Parsley	Chopped
1 package	Chopped spinach, frozen	Defrosted and drained (285-g package)
1 Omega-3 egg	Omega-3 egg white	
1 teaspoon	Salt	
115g	Yogurt cheese	(or plain yogurt)
45g	Instant oatmeal	
455g	Bison or beef, minced	
225g	Turkey, minced	
	Cooking spray	

Preheat oven to 350°F/180C°/GM4.

Heat medium-sized frying pan. Remove pan from heat, spray with cooking spray, wait a few seconds and then return to heat. When oil is hot, add onion, carrot and celery. Cook for 10 minutes over medium heat, stirring occasionally. Add garlic, cayenne pepper, thyme and parsley. Remove from heat and allow to cool.

In food processor bowl, combine spinach with eggs (whole and egg white), salt and yogurt cheese. Process until well combined. Add oatmeal and pulse until combined.

In large bowl, combine minced meats (you can use any meats you prefer – just make sure they are lean!). Add onion, carrot and celery mixture to meat. Add spinach mixture to meat. Combine well. (I use my clean wet hands, but you can use whatever you prefer – just make sure to mix well.)

On baking sheet, form meat mixture into a loaf about 6 inches wide and 3 inches high. Bake in oven until internal temperature reads 160°F/70°C, which usually takes about an hour. Remove from oven and let rest 15–20 minutes before serving.

Note: If you must glaze with ketchup, go ahead! Add 4 tablespoons ketchup painted on top of loaf. This will add 15 calories and 4 grams of carbohydrates per tablespoon of ketchup (or use one of the low-carbohydrate ketchups).

Recipe Nutritional Breakdown	Amount per Serving
Calories	314
Fat (g)	12
Saturated (g)	4
Polyunsaturated (g)	2
Monounsaturated (g)	4
Cholesterol (mg)	129
Carbohydrates (g)	13
Fibre (g)	3
Sugars (g)	0
Protein (g)	38

COMPLETE MEAL SUGGESTION

Serve with 85g steamed broccoli with fresh lemon juice and 100g cooked pearl barley.

Meal Nutritional Breakdown	Amount per Serving
Calories	436
Fat (g)	13
Saturated (g)	4
Polyunsaturated (g)	3
Monounsaturated (g)	5
Cholesterol (mg)	129
Carbohydrates (g)	40
Fibre (g)	6
Sugars (g)	0
Protein (g)	42.5

Stuffed Bell Peppers

Servings: 3 (two peppers per person)   *Degree of Difficulty: Challenging, but worth it*
Preparation Time: 30 minutes   *Time from Start to Eating: 1 hour*

Amount	Ingredients	Preparation
340ml	Chicken broth	Low-fat, low-sodium (use water or any broth, if preferred)
65g	Pearl barley	
55g	Onion	Diced
30g	Celery	Diced
35g	Carrots	Diced
1 tablespoon	Cumin	
2 teaspoons	Cayenne pepper	
½ teaspoon	Cinnamon	
45g	Mushrooms	Sliced
2 tablespoons	Olive or vegetable oil	
455g	Bison or beef, minced	
	Salt, to taste	
	Pepper, to taste	
225ml	Wine	Whatever you might have on hand is fine
3 tablespoons	Pumpkin seeds	
1 tablespoon	Cilantro	Chopped
	Seeds from 1 pomegranate*	
6	Peppers, red or green	
	Cooking spray	

*To seed a pomegranate, put the pomegranate in a bowl of water, cut it open and the seeds will float out easily.

Simmer chicken broth in small saucepan over medium-high heat, then add barley, bring to a boil, reduce heat, cover and simmer for 30 minutes until barley is tender.

Heat frying pan over medium-high heat. Remove pan from heat, spray with cooking spray, wait a few seconds and then return to heat. Add onion, celery and carrots, stirring and allowing to brown. Add cumin, 1 teaspoon cayenne and cinnamon, stirring to combine. Remove from pan and place mixture in large bowl. Add cooked barley to bowl.

In hot pan, add mushrooms, cooking over high heat until they are browned and no longer give off moisture. Remove from pan and add to bowl.

In same pan, add 1 tablespoon oil. When oil is hot, add bison. Season with salt and pepper and cook until all meat is browned. Remove meat from pan and add to bowl.

Deglaze pan by adding wine. Cook on low heat, approximately 5 minutes, until wine reduces to almost a syrup consistency. Pour over contents in bowl.

Return pan to heat. Add pumpkin seeds, 1 teaspoon cayenne and 1 tablespoon oil. Stir until seeds start to brown. Add to contents of bowl.

Preheat oven to 350°F/180°C/GM4.

Add cilantro and pomegranate seeds to bowl. Adjust seasonings.

Cut tops off peppers. Cut out membranes and remove all seeds. (If using green peppers, many people like to parboil the peppers for about 10 minutes, then shock in cold water. This takes away the sharp flavour and makes them more tender.)

Fill peppers with meat stuffing and set in casserole dish. Set tops alongside each pepper. Bake 10 to 15 minutes, until peppers are tender and filling is hot. Place tops on peppers when serving.

Optional: Pour a tin of evaporated skim milk over peppers before cooking. This adds a creaminess that some people really love. It will add 37 calories, 0.1 grams of fat and 5.4 grams of carbohydrates per serving.

Recipe Nutritional Breakdown	Amount per Serving
Calories	411
Fat (g)	12
Saturated (g)	3
Polyunsaturated (g)	4
Monounsaturated (g)	4
Cholesterol (mg)	81
Carbohydrates (g)	41
Fibre (g)	8
Sugars (g)	0
Protein (g)	36

Taco Salad

Servings: 4
Preparation Time: 15 minutes

Degree of Difficulty: Easy
Time from Start to Eating: 15 minutes

Amount	Ingredients	Preparation
55g	Onion	Chopped
1 tablespoon	Tomato paste	
1 teaspoon	Coriander	
¼ teaspoon	Cumin	
1 tablespoon	Chilli powder	
½–1 teaspoon	Cayenne pepper	(Optional)
455g	Beef, minced	
1 tin	Garbanzo beans	Drained and rinsed (425-g tin)
1 tin	Red kidney beans	Drained and rinsed (425-g tin)
1 bag	Iceberg lettuce with carrots	(or head of lettuce)
1 bag	Cabbage	Chopped
1	Avocado	Sliced and peeled
½ packet	Potato crisps	Your favourite healthy crisps
115g	Cheddar cheese	Low-fat, grated
	Cooking spray	
1 teaspoon	Salt	
	Pepper, to taste	

Heat a heavy frying pan over medium-high heat. Remove pan from heat, spray with cooking spray, wait a few seconds and then return to heat. Add onion and stir occasionally until lightly browned (5 minutes or so). Reduce heat to medium. Add tomato paste, coriander, cumin, chilli powder and cayenne pepper. Stir for about 1 minute – you should be able to smell cumin. Add minced meat. Stir occasionally until fully browned. Add 60 ml water, garbanzo beans and kidney beans. Stir for 1 minute. Add salt and pepper to taste.

In a large bowl, add lettuce, cabbage, avocado, chips and grated cheese. Toss well. Now pour minced beef and bean mixture over lettuce and toss well.

Note: Minced turkey, chicken, lean pork or buffalo can be substituted for beef. Adding the cabbage adds fibre and some good nutrition to the meal.

You can substitute black beans for kidney beans. This is also good with green and red peppers, jalapeños and chipotles.

Recipe Nutritional Breakdown	Amount per Serving
Calories	557
Fat (g)	20
Saturated (g)	5
Polyunsaturated (g)	2
Monounsaturated (g)	11
Cholesterol (mg)	90
Carbohydrates (g)	51
Fibre (g)	11
Sugars (g)	0
Protein (g)	45

SEAFOOD

Poached Salmon

Servings: 4
Preparation Time: 20 minutes

Degree of Difficulty: Easy
Time from Start to Eating: 30 minutes

Amount	Ingredient	Preparation
455g	Salmon	Bones removed, preferably with skin on

Fill a large pan two-thirds full of water. Bring to a boil, then reduce to a simmer. Add salmon, which will drop temperature of water. Keep heat on. You'll want water temperature to come back up to 190°F/88°C but not to a boil. (Boiling makes salmon rubbery.) Once water is to temperature, cover, reduce heat and leave for about 15 minutes, checking occasionally that it's not too hot or cool.

To check doneness, use a fork on flesh side of salmon. It'll flake easily with a fork when done. If you prefer more rare, you'll want it to flake less easily. Well done, it'll flake all the way down to skin when you insert a fork and twist lightly. Cook salmon until your doneness preference, remembering that it'll continue cooking a few minutes after removed from water. Remove salmon from water, put on cutting board and cover with foil, letting sit for 5 to 10 minutes.

You now have a great building block for many healthy meals and snacks, with a great source of omega-3 oils.

Recipe Nutritional Breakdown	Amount per Serving
Calories	208
Fat (g)	12
Saturated (g)	2
Polyunsaturated (g)	4
Monounsaturated (g)	4
Cholesterol (mg)	67
Carbohydrates (g)	0
Fibre (g)	0
Sugars (g)	0
Protein (g)	23

Fish Tacos

Servings: 4 (2 tacos per person)
Preparation Time: 15 minutes

Degree of Difficulty: Easy
Time from Start to Eating: 20 minutes

Amount	Ingredients	Preparation
455g	Halibut, cod, or red snapper	Filleted, then cut into strips
	Salt, to taste	
	Pepper, to taste	
8	Corn tortillas	Warmed in microwave
115g	Cabbage	Shredded
225ml	Salsa	
2	Limes	Quartered
	Cooking spray	

Preheat oven to 400°F/200°C/GM6.

Lightly season fish strips with salt and pepper. (Fish strips should be about 1 inch wide and 5 inches long.) Place on non-stick baking sheet or one that is lightly sprayed with cooking spray and put in oven. Let bake 6 minutes, then turn them over carefully so that they don't fall apart and bake 2 to 3 more minutes.

Place a warmed tortilla on a plate, one or two fish strips on top, cabbage and salsa. Lightly squeeze some fresh lime juice over taco. Fold tortilla over to serve.

Recipe Nutritional Breakdown	Amount per Serving
Calories	277
Fat (g)	5
Saturated (g)	1
Polyunsaturated (g)	2
Monounsaturated (g)	1
Cholesterol (mg)	47
Carbohydrates (g)	26
Fibre (g)	5
Sugars (g)	0
Protein (g)	34

COMPLETE MEAL SUGGESTION

Serve with 45g brown rice.

Meal Nutritional Breakdown	Amount per Serving
Calories	327
Fat (g)	5
Saturated (g)	1
Polyunsaturated (g)	2
Monounsaturated (g)	1
Cholesterol (mg)	47
Carbohydrates (g)	37
Fibre (g)	5
Sugars (g)	0
Protein (g)	35

Seared Scallops

Servings: 4
Preparation Time: 20 minutes

Degree of Difficulty: Easy
Time from Start to Eating: 30 minutes

Amount	Ingredients	Preparation
1 tablespoon	Olive oil	
1	Onion	Chopped
170g	Quinoa	
2 teaspoons	Parsley	Chopped
1 teaspoon	Thyme	Chopped
425ml	Chicken broth	Fat-free, low-sodium
1	Clove garlic	(optional)
2	Grapefruits	Peeled and sectioned (or tinned OK but not in heavy syrup)
1	Avocado	Pitted and sliced
680g	Scallops*	
1 teaspoon	Grapefruit zest	(optional)
	Cooking spray	

*Some fresh scallops still have what's known as a 'foot' – a tough muscle – attached. The foot will be a small protuberance extending from the circle shape of the scallop. Just pull off the foot by hand to clean the scallop and prepare for cooking.

Heat chicken broth in microwave.

In medium-sized saucepan, heat olive oil. Add onion and cook for 5 minutes until onion becomes translucent but not brown. Add garlic. Stir in quinoa, cook for 3 minutes, then add parsley, thyme and chicken broth and bring to a boil. Reduce to a simmer, cover and cook for 15 minutes, until quinoa is done (should be tender).

Arrange grapefruit sections with avocado slices on plates, alternating sections of grapefruit with avocado. Portion quinoa onto plates.

Heat a frying pan over medium-high heat so that it is very hot. Remove pan from heat, spray with cooking spray, wait a few seconds and then return to heat. When smoking hot, add scallops, a few at a time. Let scallops sear. After 2 minutes or so, turn over and cook on other side for 1 minute. Remove from pan. Continue this in batches.

Plate scallops and sprinkle grapefruit zest over everything.

Note: Scallops are delicious and easy to cook. The only danger is that they become quite rubbery if overcooked. And they overcook very quickly.

Recipe Nutritional Breakdown	Amount per Serving
Calories	461
Fat (g)	13
Saturated (g)	2
Polyunsaturated (g)	3
Monounsaturated (g)	7
Cholesterol (mg)	56
Carbohydrates (g)	49
Fibre (g)	5
Sugars (g)	0
Protein (g)	39

Tuna Tartare

Servings: 4
Preparation Time: 20 minutes

Degree of Difficulty: Moderate
Time from Start to Eating: 20 minutes

Amount	Ingredients	Preparation
455g	Tuna	Sushi grade, diced
3 tablespoons	Sesame seeds	
2 tablespoons	Chives	Chopped
3 tablespoons	Ginger	Diced
85g	Tomatoes	Diced
pinch	Cayenne pepper	
	Salt, to taste	
	Pepper, to taste	
1½ teaspoons	Sesame oil	
1½ teaspoons	Chili oil	(hot Asian oil)
	Ginger soy vinaigrette	
	(page 192)	

Preheat oven to 325°F/170°C/GM3.

Cover tuna with plastic wrap and keep chilled (plastic should be directly on tuna, not stretched over bowl).

Sprinkle sesame seeds onto cookie sheet and put in hot oven for 5 minutes or so, until lightly toasted. They burn easily, so keep an eye on them.

Combine tuna, chives, ginger, tomato, cayenne pepper, salt and pepper in a bowl. Stir gently. Add light drizzle of sesame oil and splash of chili oil. Very gently stir to combine again. (If you overstir, you'll start to emulsify the mixture and it won't look as nice. Taste will be the same, however.) Portion onto plates and sprinkle with toasted sesame seeds.

You can make this in small batches, tasting it as you go along to get the seasonings right.

Serve Ginger Soy Vinaigrette on the side.

Recipe Nutritional Breakdown	Amount per Serving
Calories	145
Fat (g)	2
Saturated (g)	0.5
Polyunsaturated (g)	1
Monounsaturated (g)	0.5
Cholesterol (mg)	51
Carbohydrates (g)	3
Fibre (g)	1
Sugars (g)	0
Protein (g)	27

COMPLETE MEAL SUGGESTION

Serve with whole-wheat crackers (15 or so).

Meal Nutritional Breakdown	Amount per Serving
Calories	300
Fat (g)	10
Saturated (g)	2
Polyunsaturated (g)	4
Monounsaturated (g)	3
Cholesterol (mg)	51
Carbohydrates (g)	22
Fibre (g)	4
Sugars (g)	0
Protein (g)	24

Tuna Salad (Version 1)

Servings: 2
Preparation Time: 5 minutes

Degree of Difficulty: Easy
Time from Start to Eating: 30 minutes

Amount	Ingredients	Preparation
170g	Albacore tuna packed	Rinsed and drained well in water
1 tablespoon	Sweet pickle relish	
2 tablespoons	Yogurt cheese	

Combine all ingredients in a bowl, cover and refrigerate for 30 minutes before eating.

(Again, if you think yogurt cheese is too tangy, mix it with low-fat mayonnaise or low-fat soured cream.)

Recipe Nutritional Breakdown	Amount per Serving
Calories	130
Fat (g)	3
Saturated (g)	1
Polyunsaturated (g)	1
Monounsaturated (g)	1
Cholesterol (mg)	37
Carbohydrates (g)	4
Fibre (g)	0
Sugars (g)	0
Protein (g)	21

COMPLETE MEAL SUGGESTION

Served open-faced on a wheat bran slice of toast, with a side serving of apple.

Meal Nutritional Breakdown	Amount per Serving
Calories	281
Fat (g)	4
Saturated (g)	1
Polyunsaturated (g)	1
Monounsaturated (g)	1
Cholesterol (mg)	37
Carbohydrates (g)	38
Fibre (g)	4
Sugars (g)	0
Protein (g)	24

Tuna Salad (Version 2)

Servings: 2
Preparation Time: 5 minutes

Degree of Difficulty: Easy
Time from Start to Eating: 30 minutes

Amount	Ingredients	Preparation
170g	Albacore tuna packed	Rinsed and drained well in water
2 teaspoons	Onion	Minced
2 teaspoons	Celery	Minced
2 tablespoons	Yogurt cheese	
1 tablespoon	Dill weed	
½ teaspoon	Dry mustard powder	

Combine all ingredients in a bowl, cover and refrigerate for 30 minutes before eating. (Again, if you think yogurt cheese is too tangy, mix it with low-fat mayonnaise or low-fat soured cream.)

Recipe Nutritional Breakdown	Amount per Serving
Calories	127
Fat (g)	3
Saturated (g)	1
Polyunsaturated (g)	1
Monounsaturated (g)	1
Cholesterol (mg)	37
Carbohydrates (g)	2
Fibre (g)	0
Sugars (g)	0
Protein (g)	21

COMPLETE MEAL SUGGESTION

Serve open-faced on slice of wheat bran toast with an orange.

Meal Nutritional Breakdown	Amount per Serving
Calories	261
Fat (g)	4
Saturated (g)	1
Polyunsaturated (g)	1
Monounsaturated (g)	2
Cholesterol (mg)	37
Carbohydrates (g)	32
Fibre (g)	5
Sugars (g)	0
Protein (g)	25

VEGETABLES

Ratatouille

Servings: 4
Preparation Time: 20 minutes

Degree of Difficulty: Moderate
Time from Start to Eating: 1 hour

Amount	Ingredients	Preparation
55g	Onion	Diced
3	Garlic cloves	Minced
	Salt, to taste	
	Pepper, to taste	
455g	Tomatoes	Peeled and seeded (or 455g tinned, drained)
1 tablespoon	Olive oil	
115g	Courgettes	1-inch cubes
115g	Aubergine	Peeled, 1-inch cubes
30g	Red bell pepper	Seeded, 1-inch squares
1 tablespoon	Herbs de Provence	
	Cooking spray	

Preheat oven to 375°F/190°C/GM5.

Heat a sauté pan. Remove pan from heat, spray with cooking oil, wait a few seconds and then return to heat. Then cook onions until soft and translucent but not browned. Add garlic and stir for 1 minute. Sprinkle with salt and pepper. Add tomatoes and cook uncovered until all excess moisture has evaporated. Stir often to avoid burning.

Heat another sauté pan. Remove pan from heat, spray with cooking oil, wait a few seconds, add a drizzle of olive oil and then return to heat. Sauté courgettes, aubergine and red bell pepper until just soft.

Add herbs de Provence to tomato mixture, then add sautéed vegetables. Stir to combine. Adjust seasonings and put into casserole dish. Bake for 30 minutes.

Recipe Nutritional Breakdown	Amount per Serving
Calories	85
Fat (g)	4
Saturated (g)	0.5
Polyunsaturated (g)	0.5
Monounsaturated (g)	3
Cholesterol (mg)	0
Carbohydrates (g)	12
Fibre (g)	3
Sugars (g)	0
Protein (g)	2

Roasted Butternut Squash Soup

Servings: 8   *Degree of Difficulty: Easy*
Preparation Time: 15 minutes   *Time from Start to Eating: 2 hours*

Amount	Ingredients	Preparation
pinch	Salt	
pinch	Pepper	
pinch	Nutmeg	
pinch	Cayenne pepper	
pinch	Cloves	
1	Butternut squash	Cut in half, seeds removed
115ml	White wine	Riesling or Chardonnay works well
1 tablespoon	Olive oil	
1	Onion	Chopped
3	Carrots	Chopped
3	Celery stalks	Chopped
910ml	Chicken or vegetable	Low-fat; low-sodium broth

Preheat oven to 350°F/180°C/GM4.

Lightly sprinkle salt, pepper, nutmeg, cayenne pepper and cloves on inside flesh of squash. Sprinkle some water and wine (just a splash) on a baking sheet. Lay squash face down (skin side up) on baking sheet and bake 90 minutes (check after 60 minutes, just to be sure). Test squash with a paring knife to make sure it's tender, then remove from oven and allow to cool on baking sheet.

Heat olive oil in stockpot. When oil is hot, add onion, carrots and celery, cooking about 15 minutes but not browning vegetables.

Scoop out squash into a bowl. Be careful not to allow any skin into the mix. Put baking sheet on the hob, add a little wine to the sheet, and scrape all browned bits off baking sheet. This is caramelized squash, which is full of flavour. Pour this directly into stockpot with vegetables. Add remainder of white wine and allow to cook at least 5 minutes.

Add squash to stockpot, then chicken or vegetable broth. Bring to a boil, then reduce heat so that mixture simmers for 1 hour.

Remove stockpot from heat, let cool slightly and blend soup with a hand blender until smooth. Strain through a sieve before serving. Adjust seasonings.

I like to serve it with toasted pecans, walnuts or croutons. It's low-fat, rich, creamy (with no dairy in it at all!) and delicious!

Recipe Nutritional Breakdown	Amount per Serving
Calories	91
Fat (g)	3
Saturated (g)	0
Polyunsaturated (g)	0
Monounsaturated (g)	2
Cholesterol (mg)	0
Carbohydrates (g)	13
Fibre (g)	2
Sugars (g)	0
Protein (g)	4

COMPLETE MEAL SUGGESTION

Serve with pulled pork over shredded cabbage, with 85g bulgur wheat.

Meal Nutritional Breakdown	Amount per Serving
Calories	478
Fat (g)	15
Saturated (g)	5
Polyunsaturated (g)	2
Monounsaturated (g)	7
Cholesterol (mg)	94
Carbohydrates (g)	40
Fibre (g)	9
Sugars (g)	0
Protein (g)	43

CHAPTER 11

Guidelines to Live and Eat By

One must eat to live and not live to eat.

— MOLIÈRE

There are a number of important guidelines that can really make or break your success in following *The Thyroid Diet*.

DRINK ENOUGH WATER

Even if you're eating exactly the right things and working out, if you're not getting enough water you may find it difficult, if not outright impossible, to lose weight. This is because the liver, which converts stored fat into energy, acts as a backup to the kidneys in detoxifying the body. If the kidneys are not functioning optimally because they are deprived of water, then the liver is diverted away from fat conversion and toward detoxification.

- Water helps the metabolism work efficiently.
- Water helps reduce appetite.
- Water helps skin appearance and tone.
- Water helps muscles work more efficiently.
- Water helps digestion, reduces constipation and encourages regular elimination.

Ideas about how much water you should drink depend on who you ask, but it's agreed that a minimum amount is eight 225-ml glasses a day. Some experts say that you should drink an additional 225-ml glass for every 25 pounds of weight you need to lose. So, if you are 50 pounds overweight, you should drink two more 225-ml glasses of water, for a total of 10 225-ml glasses. If it's particularly hot out or if you are exercising intensely, the American College of Sports Medicine suggests drinking even more – adding 170ml for every 15 minutes of activity. Philip Goglia, author of *Turn Up the Heat: Unlock the Fat-Burning Power of Your Metabolism*, recommends drinking 30ml of water per pound of weight. For most of us, this is substantially more than eight glasses. If you are a 11 st 6 woman, for example, that's 4½ litres a day, which is equal to 20 225-ml glasses a day. And if you are a 14 st 4 man, that's 25 225-ml glasses a day.

I know that the first few days after increasing water intake, you feel as if you're living in the lavatory. But this will settle down. As your body begins to recognize that you are finally taking in enough water, it gives up the water it's been holding on to. This is also the counter-intuitive but true theory that if you want to stop feeling bloated and retaining water, you need to drink more water! You'll know you're getting enough when your urine is pale yellow and nearly colourless. If it's darker, increase your water intake. (Keep in mind, however, that certain vitamins darken your urine, even if you're getting enough water.)

Spread out water consumption during the day as much as possible. One rule that some experts recommend is that you not drink water while you are eating. The theory is that if you are drinking water with your meal, you may be using it to help swallow food without fully chewing your food. You may want to drink a glass of water before your meal. It's even better if you can have a big glass of water with some sort of fibre (e.g. psyllium or a fibre supplement) before you eat.

There is anecdotal evidence that the stomach absorbs cold water more quickly, and that cold water may enhance fat-burning. The idea is that your body has to use extra energy to heat the cold water up close to body temperature – 37° – so this may help you burn more calories. However, there is also some thinking that cold water stimulates the appetite, and that warmer water is far easier to drink in large quantities. Since there is no real agreement, the best temperature is the one you like best and find easiest to drink. Personally, I have found that I can drink far more room-temperature water and am quite used to it this way. I buy 1-litre bottles of water with 'sports caps' and walk around all day with one of these.

GET ENOUGH FIBRE IN YOUR DIET

Fibre is essential to digestion and will optimize your weight-loss efforts. Sometimes called roughage, it is the part of plant foods that is not digestible. Fibre comes in two forms: (1) soluble, which dissolves in water and (2) insoluble, which does not. Foods that are high in soluble fibre include oats, barley, peas, beans and citrus fruits. Soluble fibre is also found in psyllium seed and oat bran. Good sources of insoluble fibre include wheat bran and certain vegetables.

- **Fibre absorbs water and helps create softer, larger stools, promoting regularity.**
- **Fibre can help prevent or minimize digestive tract problems and their consequences, like haemorrhoids, diverticular disease, irritable bowel syndrome and even rectal cancer.**
- **Fibre can slow the digestive process, preventing dramatic swings in blood sugar.**
- **Fibre can help lower cholesterol.**

There is evidence that fibre helps with weight loss. Fibre has minimal calories but can fill you up by adding bulk. When consumed with carbohydrates, it helps modulate the insulin response and normalize blood sugar. There is a fair amount of scientific support for fibre's ability to increase the feeling of fullness after you eat and reduce hunger levels. One study found that adding 14 grams of fibre per day was associated with a 10 per cent decrease in calorie intake and a weight loss of 5 pounds over 4 months.

In another study of 53 women who were moderately overweight and followed a 1,200-calorie-a-day diet over 24 weeks, half were given a fibre supplement and half received a placebo. The women given fibre had 6 grams a day to start, then 4 grams. After treatment, the fibre group lost a mean amount of 17.6 pounds versus 12.76 pounds in the placebo group.

There are some simple ways to incorporate fibre into your diet. Eat raw fruits and vegetables; they have more fibre than cooked or tinned. Dried fruits (especially dried figs) are also good sources of fibre. (Note, however, that dried fruits can be high-glycaemic, so use them with caution.)

Scan food labels for bread and cereal products listing whole grain or whole wheat as the first ingredient. Two slices of high-bran bread, for example, have 7 grams of fibre, compared to only 2 grams of fibre in white bread.

For breakfast cereal, one of the best is All-Bran. There are 90 calories in 45 grams of All-Bran, with 10.4 grams of fibre. It's not the tastiest cereal, but it's really good for you. Tart it up with a healthy serving of fruit, which adds even more fibre. Or add the cereal, some fruit and a handful of slivered almonds to plain yogurt and you have a very healthy snack.

Many nuts are high in fibre and are a source of good fats that help lower cholesterol. Almonds are one of the best nuts for you. Thirty-five grams provide 2.4 grams of fibre. I love to sprinkle a few over a serving of low-fat cottage cheese with some fruit as a snack.

Beans are a powerhouse – 170 grams of black beans, for example, provide a whopping 19.4 grams of fibre, with only 190 calories. Eighty-five grams of white beans (cannellini) have 16 grams of fibre and only 160 calories. You can also increase fibre in meat dishes by adding pinto beans, kidney beans or black-eyed peas.

Other high-fibre foods include apples, oranges, broccoli, cauliflower, berries, pears, Brussels sprouts, lettuce, prunes, carrots and potatoes.

Men younger than 50 require 38 grams of fibre a day; women need 25 grams. Men over 50 should get at least 30 grams; women at least 21 grams. The typical diet, however, includes only 10 grams of fibre a day or fewer. You'll probably have to add a fibre supplement, in addition to emphasizing fibre-rich foods. Start slow, because you need to give your intestinal system time to adjust. Adding too much fibre too quickly can cause discomfort.

Some fibre supplements to consider include:

- **Psyllium** – one study found that women who took 20 grams of psyllium before a meal ate less fat and felt full more quickly, helping with weight reduction. Psyllium husk is found in Metamucil products.
- **Guar gum** – supplements containing this dissolve with no grit or bulk into drinks.
- **Polycarbophil** – a synthetic fibre that has the filling and stool-softening effects of fibre but may not lower cholesterol or blood sugar like other fibres.

One of my favourite fibre products is Dr Levine's Ultimate Weight Loss Formula. Developed by internist Scott Levine as a weight-loss aid for his patients, the powdered formula makes a drink that contains five types of healthful fibre. It tastes fairly good. (I've tried both the chocolate and raspberry flavours and they're fine, especially compared to trying to choke down a couple of spoonfuls of psyllium husks floating around in a glass of water!) Dr Levine's formula provides 17 grams of fibre in one serving, so if you have a serving before both lunch and dinner, as he suggests, you will be getting 35 grams of fibre a day as your baseline. According to Levine, many people who use his product lose 1.5 to 3 pounds per week without doing anything else differently – a result achieved because of reduction of food intake, combined with reduced insulin resistance and blood sugar levels, due to the increased fibre in the diet. Because Levine's formula includes both soluble and insoluble fibres, it has other benefits including reduction of cholesterol. Levine says, 'The right kinds of fibre can be particularly helpful for insulin metabolism, especially in people who have even a few extra pounds around the middle. That abdominal weight gain – which drives increasing insulin levels and is the start of the whole metabolic syndrome – can be helped by high-fibre consumption.'

Important warning: If you switch from a low-fibre to a high-fibre diet, be very careful that you are taking your thyroid medicine at least an hour before eating in the morning so that your absorption is not impaired. High-fibre diets can change your dosage requirements, so 6 to 8 weeks after starting a high-fibre diet, you may wish to have your thyroid function tested.

THINGS TO EAT OR DRINK

- Eat spicy foods and peppers – capsaicin, the compound found in peppers such as cayenne and jalapeño, can stimulate metabolism (by as much as 40 per cent in the short term, according to some experts!). So pile on the peppers!
- Drink more tea – some studies have shown that people who drink 5 cups of green tea a day can burn 80 more calories over a 24-hour period. The caffeine and polyphenol compounds in the green tea can work to promote weight loss by helping the metabolism work more efficiently and by aiding the fat-burning process. Oolong and ginseng tea have also

been shown to have potential to aid in weight loss. So when you're thinking you might like to have a snack between meals, have a cup of metabolism-boosting tea instead. (But watch the caffeine levels if you are caffeine sensitive or have mitral valve prolapse.)

■ Snack on peanuts – nuts can be a healthy addition to your diet. One study showed that when people ate peanuts, they felt very satisfied and naturally decreased food consumption during the rest of the day. Despite the inclusion of extra calories, little change in body weight was observed. This was the first clinical study designed to confirm and explain a body of epidemiological data showing that nut eaters tend to have a lower body mass index (BMI) than non-nut eaters. (And no, the study wasn't published in a peanut-growers' magazine!) Researchers at Purdue University studied the effects of daily peanut consumption on dietary intake, satiety, energy expenditure and body weight. The principal investigator, Dr Richard Mattes of the US Department of Foods and Nutrition, observed that 'the high protein and fibre content in peanuts may play an important role in curbing hunger and thereby not promoting weight gain.' These findings are consistent with large population studies such as the Seventh Day Adventist Study and the Nurses' Health Study, where researchers found that most people who consumed about 30 grams of peanuts, nuts or peanut butter daily had lower BMI scores. Apparently, the researchers felt comfortable, concluding that peanuts and peanut butter satisfy hunger up to five times longer than some high-carbohydrate snacks such as rice cakes.

■ Add almonds – if you're looking to maintain a heart-healthy diet, you may want to incorporate almonds into it. A study in the journal *Circulation* reconfirmed a growing body of research that almonds may lower bad cholesterol levels and help reduce the risk of heart disease. A clinical trial found that women and men who ate about 30 grams (or a handful) of almonds each day lowered their LDL (the 'bad') cholesterol by 4.4 per cent from baseline. The study showed an even greater decrease of 9.4 per cent in LDL cholesterol in those who ate about two handfuls of almonds a day, indicating that the beneficial effect increases with consumption. The study also found that those who ate only 30-gram servings and those who ate more maintained their weight but did not gain weight.

THINGS TO CUT BACK OR ELIMINATE

- Reduce or eliminate alcohol – alcohol puts stress on your liver, which not only slows down the ability to clear toxins and burn fat but may also interfere with your body's ability to convert T4 to T3. Alcohol, at 7 calories per gram, is also entirely empty calories, with no nutritional value. Consider reducing or significantly limiting the alcohol in your diet.
- Cut back on caffeine – even in healthy people, caffeine can shift metabolism slightly, helping the push towards insulin resistance. Caffeine induces adrenaline production and may also trigger the release of insulin, both of which can result in food cravings and negative shifts in blood sugar. Nutritionist and leptin expert Byron Richards, author of *Mastering Leptin*, believes that caffeine can affect leptin timing. So instead of leptin hitting its highest level during sleep – which is optimal for weight loss – the timing is moved forward, resulting in excess cravings for carbohydrates between meals, as well as overeating at night.
- Cut down on sugary fizzy drinks, teas and juices – they are pretty much like mainlining sugar straight into your veins. You know the drill: there are 10 teaspoons of sugar in one can of cola. It's a real waste of calories and is one of the fastest ways to ensure dietary disaster. If you must have a glass of orange or other fruit juice in the morning, consider juicing it yourself (with the pulp in) so that you get some fibre and more nutritional value from it. Or if you are using prepared juice, consider diluting it with half water to help cut the sugar content. You'll still get some flavour from it, but with less of the sugar and calorie impact. One option for juice-lovers is to get unsweetened fruit juice, then add your own no-calorie sweetener. For example, I buy unsweetened cranberry juice concentrate (very foul-tasting unsweetened!), but I add Stevia and water and have a low-cal, low-carb, nutritious cranberry juice cocktail!

AVOID MOST SWEETENERS WHEN POSSIBLE

There are two basic categories of sweeteners: nutritive and non-nutritive. A nutritive sweetener has 4 calories per gram and provides energy like other simple carbohydrates. Nutritive sweeteners include white and brown table sugar, molasses, honey, maple syrup and corn syrup.

Sugar alcohols are also nutritive. These are derived from fruits or produced commercially and include sorbitol, mannitol, xylitol and maltitol. These sweeteners are thought to be metabolized somewhat more slowly than straight glucose-based sugars, but they can still affect your blood sugar. They are also known to cause abdominal discomfort in some people.

Non-nutritive sweeteners – sugar substitutes or artificial sweeteners – are calorie-free and will not influence blood sugar. These include saccharine (e.g. Sweet 'n Low), aspartame (e.g. NutraSweet/Equal) and sucralose (e.g. Splenda). There is still ongoing controversy over the safety of the various artificial sweeteners, however, because of alleged relationships with cancer, neurological problems and other symptoms including headaches, nausea, insomnia, dizziness, diarrhoea, depression, anxiety, memory loss and even vision changes.

Most natural health experts I know recommend that you stay away from aspartame. They are less adamant about saccharine and sucralose, so occasional use of these products is probably not going to be a problem for you.

There is one type of nutritive sweetener – stevia – that has no calories and because it is not a carbohydrate, it does not influence blood sugar. It comes from a plant native to Paraguay. With a glycaemic index of 0 and no calories, stevia reduces cravings for sweets. Hundreds of studies show that stevia lowers blood pressure, helps prevent oral bacteria and can even help regulate blood sugar. With no chemicals, it doesn't pose some of the concerns that aspartame and the other artificial sweeteners present.

Stevia is approximately 300 times sweeter than sugar. I love it in my tea or coffee. Stevia is also versatile and can be used in hot and cold beverages, on fruit and cereals, and as a sugar replacement in baking and cooking. I like to put a drop or two of stevia into unsweetened lemon/lime seltzer and make my own sugar-free 'soda'. And this actually counts towards my daily effort to get 2 litres or more of water! I also like to use stevia to naturally sweeten plain yogurt. If you take plain low-fat or fat-free yogurt, mix in fruit and some stevia, you have healthy, low-fat fruit yogurt without the artificial sweeteners!

Just like when you first switch to any sweetener, it takes a few days to adjust to the flavour. But once you're used to it, it satisfies your sweet cravings, and regular sugar – not to mention artificial sweeteners – will taste quite 'chemical' to you. I carry the single-serving powdered packets with me to work, restaurants and when I travel.

EAT A BIG BREAKFAST

You should aim to eat a big breakfast that contains a substantial amount of protein. In fact, aim to eat 25 per cent of your calories at breakfast. You should also eat at least 20 grams of protein at breakfast. A protein-heavy breakfast speeds up calorie-burning and gets the metabolism moving.

Some studies have shown that people eating a certain number of calories will lose weight if they eat more calories concentrated during breakfast, whereas others on the same number of calories will stay the same or even gain if they emphasize the calorie expenditure at lunch or dinner.

TRY TO EAT THREE MEALS A DAY
INSTEAD OF MULTIPLE MINI-MEALS

Did you know that just *thinking* about eating can actually trigger changes in your insulin levels and hormones that stimulate appetite? So your goal is to stop thinking about eating. (These days, I even switch off the television when they have a particularly enticing food advert, so that my hormones don't get interested!) But one of the most important ways you can stop thinking about eating is to know when you're going to eat and eat at regular intervals. If you eat on a fairly predictable schedule, you'll know when you're *not* eating, so you don't have to think about food during those times.

The controversial recommendation to eat three meals rather than grazing, or to eat five or six mini-meals, as is often suggested, comes from Byron Richards, a holistic nutritionist and author of the groundbreaking book, *Mastering Leptin*. He says:

> If 5–6 small meals a day are needed to maintain energy, the metabolic situation is not in good shape. Eating very small meals may cause some weight loss, but metabolism will likely slow down before the weight goal is achieved. Even a low-calorie snack increases insulin release, thus fat-burning mode ceases or never begins. Only by increasing the amount of time between meals will proper weight loss take place.

According to Richards, this advice to eat small, frequent meals comes from the body-building and diabetes communities. Body-builders, says Richards, can eat more times a day because they have shortened the time that their insulin levels cycle up and down by eating consistently at high-calorie levels and burning calories intensively through their muscle development. People with diabetes, according to Richards, have a malfunctioning insulin and glucagon metabolism. They have to use calories like a drug to strictly regulate insulin levels. But these examples are not necessarily applicable for the rest of us, because, according to Richards, we need to condition our liver into better responsiveness and fitness by balancing our leptin. Working towards having just three meals a day and spacing meals 5 to 6 hours apart is Richards' solution to optimizing leptin balance.

I admit that it sounded counter-intuitive to me, but in addition to his theories on leptin, there is justification for Richards' recommendation. Look at the French, who do not have nearly the obesity problem that exists in the US or, to a growing extent, in the UK. Experts studying the French diet have found that the French tend to eat three meals a day, rarely snack and take in fewer calories at a meal than most Americans. The typical slim French person is *not* having six mini-meals throughout the day.

Research studies have also found a correlation between more meals per day and obesity. Studies found that women who were obese ate one meal more per day on average than those who were not obese. The overweight women tended to eat more between-meal snacks than the women who were of normal weight.

After switching to three meals a day, I found that after a few days this approach actually worked for me and I started to notice that I felt more energetic than when I was eating lots of mini-meals. I also found that knowing the times when I would be eating made me stop thinking about what snack I could have, when I should have it and so on.

In the beginning you may still need to snack. But try cutting back to one snack a day and eventually see if you can give up your snack entirely.

EAT A LIGHTER DINNER
AND NOTHING ELSE AFTERWARDS

Dinner should be your lightest meal whenever possible. Keep in mind that most of us don't require large portions. We especially don't need a lot of starchy carbohydrates like pasta, bread, potatoes and rice. If you are going to eat starches, you're better off eating them earlier in the day when your body needs the fuel and is more likely to burn off the calories.

Byron Richards believes that we should finish eating dinner at least 3 hours before bedtime. One of his key rules to balancing leptin is 'Never eat after dinner. Allow 11–12 hours between dinner and breakfast. Never go to bed on a full stomach.'

Many experts agree with Richards that we should go to bed slightly hungry. Not so hungry or starving that hunger pangs will keep you awake, but your stomach should feel nearly empty. Your body is looking for fuel to burn during the night, and it is going to burn either undigested dinner or (what you really want) pull from your fat stores. If you go to bed with your stomach nearly empty and insulin levels low, your body is much more likely to go to your fat stores. But if you have a big meal or a large snack before bed, you have insulin flooding your system and glucose circulating that will be stored in your fat cells.

If you've skipped dinner and need a snack, it should not be more than 100 calories and should ideally include a protein and a carbohydrate. Try 55 grams of low-fat cottage cheese and a half-serving of fruit, or a small serving of high-fibre breakfast cereal with a splash of milk.

Again, there is justification for Richards' approach. In the study comparing obese women and women of normal weight, the overweight women tended to eat more food later in the day and evening than their normal-weight counterparts.

I had to get used to eating a smaller dinner and not snacking before bedtime. Before, I could easily down a dozen crackers and a piece of fruit before bed (and wake up bloated and up half a pound on the scales). But I adjusted to going to bed with an empty stomach, waking up with no bloating and with the scales showing some weight loss. It also primed me to want to eat a heartier, higher-calorie breakfast.

EAT SLOWLY AND CHEW THOROUGHLY

Your mother always said to chew your food, and she was right! Chewing thoroughly and eating slowly is important. When you chew thoroughly, you let the digestive juices in your mouth and throat do their work to properly break down and begin digesting your food. At the same time, you extend the time you're actually eating, giving your brain time to receive the 'I feel full' feeling, which takes about 10 minutes after you start eating to generate. So slow down and chew!

FOLLOW SOME BASIC FOOD-COMBINING RULES

Why and how these rules work is a book unto itself. But there are some basic food-combining principles that you may want to try. Many people report that they have much more success with their weight-loss efforts when they follow these fairly simple rules.

- Try to eat protein with non-starchy vegetables. That means you don't really want to have a baked potato with your steak. You're better off with a big salad and some sautéed mushrooms on the side.
- Avoid milk and meat at the same meal. Having milk with your meat slows down digestion.
- Eat one type of protein per meal. Don't have the beef and chicken fajita combo, or a surf-and-turf combo. Combining proteins makes them harder to digest. You can, however, add eggs to other proteins, like steak and eggs, or ham quiche.
- Don't eat fruit with meat or heavy meals, as it becomes harder to digest and can raise blood sugar.

STICK WITH YOUR PROGRAMME ON THE WEEKENDS

One study found that most people in Western countries consume more calories, fat and alcohol Friday through Sunday compared with the rest of the week. Typically, those aged 2 and older were eating 82 more calories per day on Friday through Sunday compared with Monday through

Thursday. But the biggest increase was among those 19 to 50 years old, who were taking in 115 calories more per day. Those calories tended to come more from fat and alcohol, while carbohydrates and proteins dropped. If you do this every Friday, Saturday and Sunday, those extra weekend calories could mean that every 4 months you gain more than a pound, or around 5 pounds per year! So try not to let go on the weekends!

EAT SMART WHEN YOU EAT OUT

Speaking of weekends, you may go to your favourite restaurants then. In general, we're dining out more than ever before. And this may be contributing to expanding waistlines.

It is so easy to wreak havoc on your weight-loss efforts if you're not paying attention. For example, check out these calorie counts, according to the Center for Science in the Public Interest (CSPI), a Washington, DC-based consumer group:

- Starbucks White Chocolate Mocha (570ml) made with whole milk and whipped cream has 600 calories, which is equivalent to a Big Mac.
- Nine fried mozzarella sticks, a popular appetizer at many restaurants, have 830 calories and 51 grams of fat.
- An order of kung pao chicken has 1,620 calories and 76 grams of fat.
- An order of fettuccine Alfredo contains 1,500 calories and 97 grams of fat.

So, whenever possible, choose restaurants that have healthier options. Among chain restaurants, many are recognizing the interest in healthier, lower-carbohydrate, low-fat or low-calorie food that tastes decent. For example, Subway offers several 6-inch subs with 7 grams of fat or fewer, and Pizza Hut has added a lower fat pizza and salads to its menu options.

And if you have to eat at a burger place, get a burger or chicken, take off half of the bun, get a side salad and definitely skip the fries! One order of Burger King king-sized fries (170 grams) has 600 calories and 30 grams of fat; McDonald's super-sized fries (200 grams) have 610 calories and 29 grams of fat. McDonald's and other fast-food restaurants are introducing a variety of healthier entrée salads. If you don't drown them in fatty dressings, they are better fast-food options.

KEEP TRACK OF WHAT YOU EAT

Until eating healthy foods and avoiding foods and activities that cause you to gain weight, and exercising regularly, all become habit, you can use some help. This is where tools for planning and tracking, as well as support from other people on the journey, can make or break the success of your efforts. There are many dozens of tools and options out there for you – from individual weight-loss counsellors and experts in your own area to nationally-known programmes, from simple tracking sheets to sophisticated programmes you can run on your home PC.

I've reviewed or tried many programmes but am recommending only a few that are readily available, because they are user-friendly, provide support and tools to aid you in your weight-loss effort, and are accessible to most people around the world.

One of the most powerful things you can do is *write things down*. Studies have shown that people who write down everything they eat can actually lose weight, even if not formally dieting, simply because the act of writing it down makes them more aware and likelier to make better choices. Write down your goals. Plan what you're going to eat. Keep track of calories, carbs, fat, water or other nutrients, and exercise hours, intensity or calories burned.

There are special books and journals you can buy for this purpose. One particularly good diary is the *Fat Tracker Daily Diary*, from Karen Chisholm. See www.thefattracker.com for more information. You can also use a notepad, your computer, a calendar, or a loose-leaf binder. It doesn't matter what form your journal takes; it's the action of sitting down and thinking about your goals, what you're going to eat and assessing what you've eaten that makes the difference.

To get you started, I've included simple tracking sheets in Chapter 9 that you can photocopy and use to keep track of your food, exercise and supplement intake. Other sites and tools are also in this section, and are featured at www.goodmetabolism.com. If you want a more formalized way to keep close track of your nutritional intake, emotions and fitness, there are some tools I'd highly recommend.

DietPower

DietPower is a software programme that nutritionally analyses the foods you've eaten, calculates your calorie intake along with dozens of different nutrients, and keeps track of the calories burned in various exercises and fitness activities. The programme even keeps track of proper water intake and is entirely customizable in terms of your target ratios of fats, carbs and proteins, for example. One of the most unique aspects of DietPower is its ability to 'learn' your metabolism. It monitors your metabolism and adjusts daily calorie targets in recognition of your unique metabolic rate while tracking your intake of 33 nutrients, calories burned in exercise, and water intake. It is not a diet or a programme that tells you what to eat; it is a tool that shows you what you've eaten and evaluates your metabolism. A free downloadable trial version lets you test this tool to see if it's a good fit for you.

Ediets and Weight Watchers Online

Both of these diet powerhouse sites have capabilities to keep track of what you eat, how much and your exercise and fitness. Ediets, with multiple diet approaches to choose from – for example, Atkins, low-fat, diets for people with diabetes – has more options in terms of the overall food approach. Weight Watchers, with its point programme, is somewhat less flexible, because it doesn't differentiate between carbs and protein, for example, in assigning points. Overall calories, fat and fibre are mainly used to calculate the point value of a food. But the points programme is a very easy way to keep track of things, and if you use their programme but choose low-glycaemic foods over higher-glycaemic carbohydrates, the points approach can be a useful tracking device. Weight Watchers also has a very easy-to-learn interface. I tried the site and within about 15 minutes had my targets and point calculations for the day already entered and I was navigating with ease. Ediets, with more options and permutations, is not quite as simple to navigate but is rich with content and information.

Physique Transformation Program's Personal Food Analyst

One unique tracking tool available only online is the Physique Transformation Program's Personal Food Analyst, or PFA. The PFA has a vast database of many thousands of foods – everything from fast foods to restaurant specialities to supermarket brands are here. According to your own or the programme's goals for various nutrients and food components such as protein, fat and carbs, the programme gives you a letter grade – A+, A, B+, B and so on, down to F – based on how you did for the day compared to your goals. This approach is particularly appealing, inspires the competitive aspect in many people, and is easy to understand.

PLAN WHAT YOU'RE GOING TO EAT AND BUY

When it comes to planning, Physique Transformation's Personal Food Analyst will let you enter foods and exercise in advance so that you can essentially plan out ahead of time what you will eat and what exercise you will do. If you select the right foods, shooting for an A rating from the programme, then follow your own plan, you can guarantee that you'll eat well. The Personal Food Analyst doesn't tell you what to eat, however, so you will need to come up with your own ideas and make your own choices.

Ediets and Weight Watchers online really shine for those who want it all planned out – even to the extent of generating an automatic shopping list. You can pick out menus you like – many options in both programmes include frozen low-calorie meals and other convenience foods or fully-cooked gourmet meals – for an entire week and get the menus and recipes printed out, along with shopping lists. If you don't want to have to plan anything, these approaches may be right for you.

Weight Watchers also has a really useful feature called Recipe Builder, which lets you enter a recipe and get a Weight Watchers point count for it. You can then modify ingredients and preparation techniques to make the recipe healthier and reduce the point count.

GET SUPPORT FROM OTHERS

When it comes to weight loss, some of us are social animals and do better when we're in a support group. One study looked at more than 500 people, half of whom were doing a self-help weight-loss programme and half who were doing a commercial weight-loss programme. After 2 years, about 150 people from each group were still continuing. The self-help group lost about 3 pounds in a year on average, then gained it back during the second year. In contrast, the commercial group – those going to Weight Watchers – maintained a weight loss of around 10 pounds in the first year, and after the second year concluded they were still an average of 6 pounds lighter than when they'd started. Those who went to even more Weight Watchers sessions did better than those who attended fewer sessions.

If you find in-person support and camaraderie essential, consider joining a group like Weight Watchers. Local hospitals frequently offer weight-loss support groups, and some companies even encourage employees to organize weight-loss groups or lunchtime walking programmes for weight loss.

If group support is not your style, you may prefer more of a one-on-one counselling approach. You have several options. You can work with a dietician, nutritionist or therapist who has a compatible style and philosophy to your own. This may sound expensive, but in the long run it's comparable to what you'd end up paying for some of the more costly commercial weight-loss centres that offer one-on-one counselling and you won't have the pressure to buy products or supplements. Plus, you'll have much more customized support from highly trained experts, rather than a 'one-size-fits-all' diet programme and support from folks who are not typically expert in physiology, nutrition, weight loss or cognitive behaviour, although they are trained to help you implement their company's programme.

Finally, more and more people are turning to online support communities, ranging from the more formalized weight-loss communities at places like Ediets, Weight Watchers Online and Physique Transformation, to AOL's numerous weight-loss and diet chat rooms – informal places like my own Thyroid Diet & Weight Loss Support Forum. There are thousands of interactive forums, bulletin boards, chats, list servs and other interactive online support activities available 24 hours a day. The key is to find the community that has the types of support you need when you need it. If you're looking for a range of support, one of the bigger sites, like Ediets or Weight Watchers Online, might be a good choice, because you'll find support communities focused on different approaches, different amounts of weight to be lost, fitness issues, and numerous expert chats where you can ask questions from counsellors and experts. Basically, you'll find a great deal of variety in terms of support offered. If you have diabetes and are following a gluten-free diet to try and lose weight, for example, you'll want to find a specialized support group of others in the same situation.

PART 5

Moving Forward

CHAPTER 12

What to Do After You've Tried Everything

When nothing seems to help, I go look at a stonecutter hammering away at his rock perhaps a hundred times without as much as a crack showing in it. Yet at the hundred and first blow it will split in two, and I know it was not that blow that did it, but all that had gone before.

— JACOB RIIS

There may be a point when you truly have tried everything you can on your own and have given time and dedication to your weight-loss effort with no success. Before you say you've done everything, ask yourself if that is true deep down, because only you know if you have really tried or if you haven't stuck with it long enough, or if you've cut corners or been half-hearted in any way.

But when you can honestly say that you've tried it all and done it all and nothing is working, that's the point you may want to give up entirely and decide that you're never going to lose weight. Before you defrost that chocolate cheesecake in your freezer and throw yourself a pity party – don't give up! Even when you think you've tried everything, there are still more things you can do!

SPECIALIZED APPROACHES

There are a number of specialized approaches you can try. These different approaches attempt to see how you can lose weight or assess your unique metabolism to identify the best diet for you, or raise your metabolism before attempting to move you into fat loss. Some of these approaches are only meant for short-term assessment purposes; others are longer-term options.

Atkins Fat Fast

If you aren't losing any weight on your diet, the late Dr Robert Atkins recommends in *Dr Atkins' New Diet Revolution* that you go on a 'Fat Fast'. This may be a worthwhile approach to try if no diet seems to be working for you.

It involves a 1,000-calorie-per-day diet that consists of 75 to 90 per cent fat. Because very minimal protein and carbohydrates – which convert to glucose – are being provided, the body is forced into a state of lipolysis, or fat-burning, and the body's stores of fat start to burn off. According to Atkins, since carbohydrates and most proteins convert to energy by way of glucose, when you eliminate almost everything but fat from your diet, you can force even the most resistant body into a state of lipolysis.

On this diet, Atkins recommends eating five meals a day of approximately 200 calories each. Some high-fat meals could include, for example:

- 1 ounce of macadamia nuts
- 2 ounces of cream cheese or Brie
- 1 ounce of tuna or chicken salad with mayonnaise and a quarter of an avocado
- Two devilled eggs with mayonnaise
- 2 ounces of high-fat pâté

Atkins suggests trying this approach for 4 to 5 days and, if you lose weight, consider this a starting point. You can then slowly adjust by including more protein and less fat, increase calories up to 1,200 and eat four 300-calorie meals per day. If you continue to lose weight, continue shifting from fat to protein while keeping carbohydrates low. For specifics, see *Dr Atkins' New Diet Revolution*.

Curves' Metabolic Tune-up

The Curves fitness centers' founder, Gary Heavin, offers in his book *Curves: Permanent Results Without Permanent Dieting*, a different approach for people who simply are not losing weight on his diet programme. He recommends a metabolic tune-up. The point of a metabolic tune-up is not to lose weight but to increase metabolism and raise the number of calories eaten and burned per day. According to Heavin, at the end of the tune-up, your weight will be the same but your metabolism will be increased.

The metabolic tune-up approach involves the following steps:

1. **Start by weighing yourself. Your current weight is considered your 'low' weight.**
2. **Start eating a normal and healthy diet, but make sure you are eating 2,500 to 3,000 calories a day.**
3. **Weigh yourself every morning before you eat breakfast.**
4. **When you have gained 3 to 5 pounds (usually within a few days), mark that weight as your 'high' weight and stop eating a high-calorie diet.**
5. **Return to an intensive fat-burning diet.**
6. **Your goal is to stay between your low and high weights. Eat normally and higher calorie until you reach your high weight, then go back to your more intensive fat-burning diet until you get back to your low weight.**

According to Heavin, in the beginning you'll be dieting more days than you are eating normally at the higher-calorie rate. But over time, as your metabolism becomes more accustomed to the food, it will take longer to gain back the extra pounds. When you can eat for 3 to 4 weeks at the higher-calorie level without gaining weight, and are on a more intensive fat-burning diet no more than 2 days a month, then you can go back to a weight-loss programme.

Heavin's book also features a number of helpful suggestions regarding exercise, including a terrific in-home workout.

Physique Transformation Program

The online Physique Transformation Program, with its Personal Food Analyst, takes the approach that low-calorie eating makes your body an extremely efficient fat-storing machine. After a low-calorie diet, when you return to eating regular amounts, your body is so sure that you are starving that it continues to store fat aggressively, making it easier to gain weight than ever before. Programme founders Ric Rooney and Bart Hanks bring a body-building and nutritional perspective to their Physique Transformation Module, which determines your current caloric intake, identifies an optimal rate, then slowly and very systematically raises your caloric intake over time to the level needed to maximize metabolism – a process they call metabolic conditioning. Only after metabolic conditioning, which can last weeks or months, do you shift into fat-burning, weight-loss mode, where calorie levels are rotated up and down to generate loss of fat. Rooney and Hanks claim that rigorous adherence to their programme will ultimately result in burning off 2 pounds of fat per week. And they stress that the way their system is precisely structured, the weight lost is fat, not valuable muscle.

Their programme emphasizes very precise targets for nutrition and, after entering your food each day online, you are given a score ranging from A+ to F, based on whether you have met calorie and nutritional goals and not exceeded your intake of certain components such as fat and sodium. For the best results, you have to eat within a few calories of your targets each and every day, getting those calories from the proper ratios of protein, carbohydrates and fats. When you move into the fat-burning phase of the programme, caloric intake drops and you have caloric goals and ratios of protein/carbs/fat that change up and down in a lower range daily – a way to fool your metabolism, so to speak, and keep it from resetting itself permanently to accommodate fewer calories.

Physique Transformation has a number of devoted followers. You don't need to be a body-builder to do the programme, but it is not for the faint of heart. I found the programme very intriguing and got through the analysis stage and 2 weeks of metabolic conditioning. While you're not supposed to gain more than a few pounds during that process – and, according to Rooney, many people who are overweight actually lose weight – the only way to reach the caloric targets was to eat substantial amounts of low-fat carbohydrates such as potatoes and pasta. I started gaining weight quickly. When I had gained nearly 7 pounds, I knew that I could not continue with the metabolic conditioning. Despite being a Physique Transformation dropout myself, I have met many satisfied and devoted participants, including some who are hypothyroid. Ultimately, the idea that you need to eat to raise metabolism is a very sound one, and the programme emphasizes a nutritionally balanced diet. If you are not insulin resistant or carbohydrate sensitive, this may be a good option to try. The initial analysis phase is free.

Metabolic Typing

Metabolic typing is described at length in *The Metabolic Typing Diet* by William Wolcott and Trish Fahey. The basic premise of metabolic typing is that each of us has a metabolism that falls predominantly into one of three categories: carbo types, protein types, or mixed types. Carbo types do best on a diet that emphasizes carbohydrates. Protein types function best on a higher-protein diet. And mixed types can eat a diet that combines both in a balanced mix.

The book features a detailed questionnaire that you fill out to determine what sort of metabolism you have, including an assessment of whether you are a fast or slow oxidizer – a measure of your ability to metabolize fats and your reliance on carbohydrates or proteins. It also looks at how all this interacts with your nervous system, to categorize you into one of nine different metabolic types. Detailed lists of foods are provided that can supposedly stimulate, strengthen and support your particular metabolic type.

A more detailed online assessment tool for metabolic typing is available from Healthexcel.com and can be administered through Dr Joseph Mercola's practice, as well as other nutritionists and practitioners (see Appendix A). I went through this metabolic typing questionnaire, which took about an hour. The programme determined that I am a protein type and provided a variety of other details, as well as a detailed diet plan, followed by a personal phone consultation with one of Dr Mercola's trained staff members. I have incorporated many of these recommendations into my own personal dietary approaches and have found them helpful.

Mercola's No-Grain Diet

For a healthier, more rigorous version of the Atkins diet, consider looking into Dr Mercola's no-grain diet. His approach is outlined on his website, Mercola.com, and specifically in his book *The No-Grain Diet: Conquer Carbohydrate Addiction and Stay Slim for Life.*

Dr Mercola is a believer in metabolic typing, and his diet is based on the assumption that the vast majority of the overweight are carbohydrate sensitive. Mercola's approach is low-glycaemic, and limiting grains and sugars intensively is the crux of his programme. He also suggests focusing on organic, hormone-free produce and meats as often as possible. In addition, Mercola believes that most popular meats are too high in fat and advocates the use of bison/buffalo and ostrich for their quality of protein and lower fat. Rounding out Mercola's approach are recommendations regarding sleep, hydration, exercise, good fats, sunlight exposure and emotional health.

Some people who lose weight on the low-carbohydrate Atkins approach but who are concerned about how much fat they are eating may find Dr Mercola's approach healthier, with his focus on low-fat, toxin-free proteins, and on vegetables.

NUTRITIONAL CONSULTATION

If you aren't getting results on your own, it may be time to schedule some sessions with a nutritional consultant, dietician or holistic practitioner with expertise in nutrition. Not only can a nutritional consultant run the tests that can assess you for nutritional, hormonal and digestive imbalances, but a consultant can help you sort out your options to increase your odds of landing on the right approach for you.

Dana Laake, one of Washington, DC's premier preventative and therapeutic nutritionists, was asked at a women's health conference what she thought about popular diets such as the Atkins diet and Barry Sears' Zone diet. These diets have been criticized by conventional doctors as radical, too high-protein, not low-fat enough for weight loss, or not balanced enough. Dana gave excellent advice:

> No one diet is necessarily right for you. But if you're not
> losing weight eating the way you're eating now, change the
> way you're eating. You can try one of these diets and see if it
> has an effect. Then, starting there, you can work your way
> back toward a healthier, balanced version of that diet.

This is excellent advice. Conventional low-fat diets will help some people lose weight. High-fibre diets may be the key for some. Protein may be the answer for others.

Take a look at whatever way of eating you're following now, and if it isn't working, try something very different, perhaps even radical, to see if that has an effect. Once you determine that a vegetarian, non-dairy, low-glycaemic, high-fibre, high-protein, gluten-free or other diet in its purest form might be effective, you can work with a nutritionist to find a healthier, more balanced version of that diet that works best for you.

PRESCRIPTION WEIGHT-LOSS DRUGS

By now, you know that there is no magic pill that will allow you to eat unhealthy, fatty, sugary or starchy foods to your heart's content while you still lose weight. There are, however, some medications that may, as a last resort, help with weight loss. But these drugs are approved for use only alongside lifestyle modifications like controlled diet and exercise. Your doctor is not going to hand over a prescription for a weight-loss drug and tell you to go out there and strap on the feedbag! So you will have to focus on healthy eating – in some cases a low-fat diet – *before* you start looking at these drugs as options. Even then, keep in mind that weight lost on diet drugs is almost always regained when you stop taking the drug – and most people cannot remain on weight-loss drugs for life.

So in the end, weight-loss drugs are a quick fix. They may help jump-start weight loss after a long plateau, but they are not going to return you to a healthy weight and keep you there for life. Ultimately, you still need to figure out how to rebalance your metabolism, optimize your thyroid, incorporate an exercise programme and determine what combination and quantities of protein, carbohydrates and fats allow you to function your best and maintain a healthy weight.

Here is a look at one of the prescription weight-loss drugs available. Note that other drugs are sold online by unscrupulous companies offering prescriptions requiring minimal health information and no medical examination. You should *not* purchase diet drugs this way, particularly because there are a variety of potential side-effects that can be dangerous. Your health needs to be thoroughly evaluated before prescribing diet drugs, and your response to the drugs must be monitored on an ongoing basis by a doctor. If you order the drugs directly, you are bypassing this important – even lifesaving – step.

Topiramate (Topamax)

Topiramate (brand name Topamax) is an anti-epileptic drug. Topiramate helps control seizures by altering chemical impulses in the brain. In 2002, researchers began to publish studies about using topiramate for weight loss. The manufacturer, Ortho-McNeil Pharmaceuticals, sponsored one of these studies. Supporting the research by Ortho-McNeil, physicians who were studying topiramate's effects on epileptic patients noticed a trend in weight loss as a side-effect.

In one study about the weight changes in patients during clinical trials for topiramate, researchers found that a daily dose of 200mg resulted in a 5 per cent or greater weight loss in 28 per cent of the patients and 57 per cent of those treated with 800mg/day. The amount of weight lost was proportional with baseline body weight; therefore, the higher the initial body weight, the more weight the patients lost. Interestingly, those who took valproic acid, an anticonvulsant, prior to participating in the topiramate clinical trial lost even more weight. These studies were announced at an annual American Epilepsy Society Meeting in December 2002.

In 2003, two more studies were published about topiramate and weight loss. The Ortho-McNeil study, published in the *American Journal of Psychiatry*, announced that topiramate may be useful among binge eaters. The study described how topiramate prescribed for mood disorders caused patients who binge eat to do so less often. Among patients treated with topiramate for epilepsy, weight loss and loss of appetite were noted. The study included 61 patients with binge-eating disorders and obesity. For 14 weeks, one group took a flexible dose of 25–600mg topiramate each day; the other took a placebo. The topiramate group had a 94 per cent reduction in binge eating. Also, patients taking topiramate lost an average of 13 pounds. In addition to losing weight, patients' blood pressure and triglyceride levels decreased.

From the evidence in these studies, it appears that topiramate is a promising drug for weight loss and binge-eating disorders. The side-effects most often cited by study participants were headaches, tickling/prickling sensation, drowsiness and difficulty with concentration.

CHAPTER 13

Keeping the Faith

Whether you think you will succeed or not –
you're right.

– HENRY FORD

How do you keep the faith, maintain the hope that you will be able to find the right approach, stick with it, lose the weight and keep it off? It requires a combination of time, the right attitude and a bit of forward thinking.

PUT YOURSELF FIRST

Whatever new way of eating you choose, you are going to have to push yourself up higher on your own priority list. I know that I am much more likely to do just about anything – work, favours for friends, answering emails, playing with my daughter – than jump on my treadmill, because everything else seems so much more urgent.

But how much more important and urgent are everyone else's needs versus your own health and self-esteem? So make time for yourself – time to plan and shop for healthy foods, cook meals, exercise, reduce your stress – and don't be so quick to donate your valuable time to everyone and everything else when one of the most worthy causes of all is looking at you in the mirror!

PHRASE YOUR GOALS POSITIVELY

Think about your goals positively. Phrase them in your mind without using a negative word. In yoga, making a resolution is called a *shankalpa*. In yoga practice, you must always phrase your shankalpa positively in order for success. So instead of 'I need to lose weight,' focus on 'I will eat more healthily and get more exercise so that I can get to a better weight for me.'

I don't know why this works, but it does. Perhaps instead of challenging your body to a duel and telling it you are going to take something away, you are saying that you will be adding good things to it, improving it and making it better.

Patricia is going into her weight-loss efforts with the right attitude:

> I'm working with the diet and even with the changes I've made (even though I've made some mistakes) I am feeling more 'clear' and it seems my hunger is more satisfied, if you know what I mean. When I'm hungry, it's as if I have control over the hunger rather than feeling as if I *have* to eat *now*. I'm looking forward to feeling better, even if I don't lose weight. If the weight (50 lb) comes off as well, well what a *plus* that will be!

REALIZE THAT IT'S NOT A DIET – IT'S LIFE!

Don't view your change in eating habits as a diet that you can go on and off. This is life. This is hypothyroidism. This is not where you lose the extra couple of pounds, then it'll be easy to keep it off. You're on a journey and you may arrive at a target weight, but that's not your destination, because you need to change your way of eating and step up your physical activity for life. As you age, you need to adjust for the slowdown of metabolism by increasing your activity level. You can rail against this reality, or you can accept it as part of life, work it in as best as you can, and move on to living well and finding a healthy weight.

Remember the 90/10 rule. If you're doing what you're supposed to be doing 90 per cent of the time, then there are times when you can stray from the path. You have to eat a piece of birthday cake on your birthday! Some stuffing at Christmas. Just get back to your regular way of eating the next day!

DEFEAT NEGATIVE THINKING

Nutritional and weight-loss coach and therapist Dr Dave Junno feels that negative thinking can really put a damper on efforts to lose weight. According to Junno, many of us go around saying, 'I can never give up the foods I love,' or 'I can't do an exercise programme.' Or if we've tried to change our diet or tried to exercise more and haven't been successful, then we might say, 'I tried that and it hasn't worked,' or 'I don't have the discipline or the willpower.'

According to Junno, this creates a self-defeating cycle. Our negative thinking leads to inaction, which leads to no results, which confirms and reinforces the negative thinking. 'It is like we have given ourselves a life sentence without parole,' says Junno. His suggestion is to introduce one word into your vocabulary when you talk about your weight-loss efforts: *yet*.

- 'I haven't been able to give up the foods I love ... yet.'
- 'I can't do an exercise programme ... yet!'
- 'I tried that and it hasn't worked ... yet.'
- 'I don't have the discipline or willpower ... yet.'

Junno says:

> This may sound like a small step, but it opens up big possibilities. It introduces the potential for success, which can help keep us motivated to continue trying. In the future all things are possible. Anyway, how do we know we can never stay with a diet or exercise programme? Where is it written that this is impossible? Others have made these changes. Why can't we? Sure it may take work, but that doesn't mean it can't be done. Just because we haven't done it so far doesn't mean we won't be able to eventually. Many people who succeed at making healthy lifestyle changes at first experienced some failures.

Junno also suggests that we keep in mind the many things we were unsuccessful at doing the first time we tried but were eventually able to master:

> Remember riding a bike? Did you ride perfectly the first time? Probably not. Chances are you needed to practise a number of times, or build up your confidence, or just be in the right frame of mind to be willing to try.

I love the idea of holding on to the power of the word *yet*. I was a smoker from my late teens until my early 30s, and I must have stopped and started smoking a dozen times. I finally decided that all my attempts weren't failures. Instead, I was practising and eventually I would get so good at it that I would successfully stop smoking for ever. And I did! I didn't use a smoking cessation programme. I just went on straight willpower, along with a number of things I'd learned about myself in all my previous attempts. I have viewed my weight-loss efforts over the past 10 years in a similar way. I'm learning what works and what doesn't work in my own efforts to optimize my thyroid and maintain a healthy weight. And the times that things haven't worked – well, those weren't failures; they were practice! I may still have some more weight to lose, but I'm working on it. Right now, I'm not at the exact weight, body mass index and clothing size I want to be … yet! But I've finally figured out how to get there, slowly and surely. And you can, too!

HAVE HOPE FOR FUTURE DEVELOPMENTS

One thing to be encouraged about is, since there are so many overweight, frustrated people in the world, finding solutions has become a major priority for the scientific community. Tremendous research efforts are looking at various weight-loss drugs and approaches. And many new developments and drugs are in the works. Here is a brief look at some of the things you're likely to hear about in the future.

Surgeries and Devices

Implantable devices, much like pacemakers, may be able to regulate hunger signals by delivering various stimuli to the stomach lining and triggering different hormonal reactions.

C75

C75 is a drug that has been shown in animal studies to suppress appetite and burn fat. It might allow dieters to feel full on less food while burning excess fat stores. Mice that received abdominal injections of C75 in addition to a high-calorie diet burned about 33 per cent more calories and lost 50 per cent more fat than mice that did not receive the drug. Overall, the drug led to a sustained weight loss of about 20 per cent of body mass with just a moderate reduction in food intake.

Rimonabant

Rimonabant, a drug that blocks the hunger-inducing effects of marijuana, may become a new diet drug. Apparently, marijuana stimulates areas of the hypothalamus, which then releases the message that the body needs food. Rimonabant locks into the brain's receptors and prevents the body from receiving the 'feed me' messages from the body's own cannabinoids, which act like marijuana to stimulate appetite. In a 16-week trial, obese patients on the highest dose of the drug lost almost 10 pounds.

Zonisamide

When combined with a reduced-calorie diet, the epilepsy drug zonisamide may help to generate significant weight loss. One Duke University study found that participants who took zonisamide daily for 16 weeks lost an average of nearly 13 pounds, compared with about 2 pounds in patients taking placebo pills. Both groups composed mainly of women over 200 pounds also ate 500 fewer calories daily in a diet monitored by a dietician and were encouraged to increase their activity levels.

Axokine

Axokine is a drug based on a chemical in the brain that keeps injured neurons from dying. Axokine docks at a similar cell receptor in the hypothalamus as leptin, and some experts think that it fools the brain into forgetting that you've eaten fewer calories. Preliminary studies showed that people over 220 pounds (15 st 10) taking Axokine lost an average of 4.7 per cent of their weight, or 10.4 pounds, over 12 weeks, while those on a placebo actually gained a pound. Forty-eight weeks after stopping treatment, the people who took Axokine had lost an average of 12.4 pounds, or 5.6 per cent of their weight. Unfortunately, wider trials showed that Axokine may not perform much better than a placebo over time, and patients may develop resistance to the drug. Makers still have it on the drawing board.

Growth Hormone

It seems not a day goes by that we don't hear some new development about the linkage between growth hormone and weight loss. In one study, small doses of growth hormone given to people who were 40 per cent overweight generated weight loss of around 5 pounds. Researchers believe growth hormone may be promising as an obesity treatment because it helps control appetite and makes metabolism more efficient.

KB-141

KB-141 is a compound that has shown promise in animal studies. In fact, monkeys given the hormone-like compound lost 7 per cent of their body weight in just 1 week. Experts are now working on developing a drug from KB-141. KB-141 works on the same principle as the thyroid. Like thyroid hormone it helps boost metabolic rate, but without affecting heart rate. Animals given the drug had reduced cholesterol levels and reduced body weight without a faster heartbeat. Professor John Lazarus, the president of the British Thyroid Association, has said that the finding was 'very exciting'.

Nastech PYY 3-36 Spray

Another product that is in the testing phase is a nasal spray that delivers PYY for the treatment of obesity. PYY is a hormone naturally produced by the stomach in relation to the calorie content of a meal. According to results from a study conducted in 2003, obese or non-obese patients given a 90-minute intravenous infusion of PYY consumed on average 30 per cent fewer calories. All the people studied experienced a significant decrease in their overall 24-hour calorie intake. Furthermore, obese patients were observed to have lower levels of circulating PYY. Therefore, increasing levels of PYY may be an effective therapeutic strategy in treating obesity, and the nasal formula has been shown to deliver sufficient amounts of PYY for therapeutic value.

Ginseng Berry

Ginsenoside re, which is an extract from the ginseng berry, is another compound that has shown promise as both a diabetes and weight-loss treatment. Researchers from the University of Chicago's Tang Center for Herbal Medicine Research reported that daily injections of ginseng berry extract restored normal blood sugar levels in diabetic mice. Blood glucose levels fell from 222mg/dl (quite high for a mouse) to 137mg/dl (normal) within 12 days. Treated mice also had better scores on a glucose tolerance test. The extract caused the obese diabetic mice to lose more than 10 per cent of their body weight in 12 days. Untreated mice gained weight during the 12-day period. The treated mice ate 15 per cent less and were 35 per cent more active than untreated mice. Researchers are hard at work trying to develop a drug that will work similarly in humans.

Other Drugs

Researchers are also hard at work trying to apply all the latest findings about ghrelin, leptin, resistin and neuropeptide Y, the various hormones and chemicals that may lead to new weight-loss drugs. Many companies are trying to find the right combinations and drugs that will unlock the key to successful weight loss. Billions of dollars are to be made by the companies that develop safe, effective weight-loss drugs, so a tremendous amount of research is going on all the time. Stay tuned, because it's likely that something new that may be of help to thyroid patients is just around the corner!

BELIEVE IT CAN BE DONE!

For more than a decade, the US National Weight Control Registry, a collaboration between the University of Colorado and the University of Pittsburgh, has maintained a database of more than 2,000 people who have successfully lost at least 30 pounds and kept it off. The registry has found that:

- The most popular form of exercise for these weight-losers is walking.
- More than 50 per cent of those in the database did not participate in a formal weight-loss programme. Instead, they employed a lot of personal discipline.
- The average registrant has lost 60 pounds and kept it off for 5 years.

Don't buy into the doom-and-gloom statistics about weight loss or about thyroid disease. It's hard to lose weight, but it's not impossible. You can do it and *The Thyroid Diet* will help!

Perhaps the best thing is for you to hear the inspirational words of your fellow thyroid patients. Kelli had to call round to interview doctors to find the right one to help her diagnose her thyroid problem:

> You were right! It's tough to find the right one. But I found one in my area. And I think she is learning from the information I have shared with her. I was strong in my approach. The blood tests came back clearly indicating that I was hypothyroid, and I asked to be put on medication, which is working wonders. I asked for follow-up blood tests just this last week, after being on the medication for only 6 weeks, and it is working! My joints no longer are painful and I am starting to lose weight, and my depression is lifting. It's like a miracle.

Until being diagnosed with thyroid cancer in 2000, Karenna describes herself as a 'size 8 with bundles of energy':

> I didn't exercise, but could run up four flights of stairs without missing a beat. After the removal, my weight ballooned from 130 pounds [9 st 4] to 175 pounds [12½ st]. It took 3 years to take off 20 pounds. Currently I have reduced my carb intake. I did not do a full-scale low-carb, high-fat diet. I eat protein for breakfast, salad for lunch, and protein with a light salad or fruit for dinner. I steer clear of all sugar, flour, etc. It seems to work for me. I now weigh around 155 pounds [11 st 1]. I have more energy and seem to fit proportionately in my clothes better. People notice that I have lost weight and look healthier. It is a constant struggle. My former thyroid doc told me I was depressed and I should eat a more balanced diet and exercise more. How to exercise when you can hardly lift your head off the pillow is beyond me. My new thyroid doc (love him!) understands that losing weight isn't easy. He even tells me I look great the way I am!

Some readers have found their own way to weight loss. For example, Mandy has found that Weight Watchers is helping her:

> I've lost almost 20 pounds in 9 weeks and it has been a very comfortable process. I only needed to lose about 15 pounds to begin with. It is a very healthy way to lose weight. You can eat anything, so there are no cravings. One simply has to be mindful of healthy choices and proportions.

Susan found the low-glycaemic approach helpful:

> Three years ago I bought *The G-Index Diet* book by Richard Podell, on a recommendation from your website. I have been on a low-glycaemic-index diet ever since and it has been a miracle. Nothing else worked since I was diagnosed with hypothyroidism 15 years ago and, having not broken this diet

once in 3 years, my earlier failed attempts were obviously *not* due to a lack of willpower! I lost 60 pounds over the course of 15 months and, while gaining 10 pounds back, I have stabilized at a size 14 as opposed to a 20.

Jane wrote to me recently. She said she had tried different eating plans and nothing had worked ...

... until now. I've lost 10½ pounds in about two months since starting your diet. I'm also working out at Curves (for the past six months) and have reduced 20 inches but wasn't dropping real weight. The weight wouldn't come off for anything until I started this diet. It's perfect for my thyroid disorder, which started out as Graves' disease. I was very sick until I was finally diagnosed. Eventually I took the radioactive iodine and since 1989 I had gained 110 lb [7 stone 12]. I am 50 years old now and had been prepared to gain some weight with my age, but that was just too much. Before I couldn't lose more than 8 pounds and always gained it back. Six months ago I was at 240 [17 st 2]; now I'm 229.5 [16 st 5½]. I know the resistance exercise at Curves has helped me in many ways, but the weight loss is definitely from this diet. Believe me – I've learned enough about my own body to know what is and isn't going to work.

Ellen, age 36 and the mother of two, works part-time as an exercise instructor and personal trainer. At 5'9", she's a size 10 and explains how she has kept her weight in control despite her own thyroid condition:

What are my recommendations as a thyroid patient and as a fitness professional?

- At *least* three aerobic workouts per week (more if you can) and some activity every day.
- Two challenging total-body strength-training workouts per week – nothing boosts your metabolism like additional muscle!

- Smaller more frequent meals (five or six mini-meals per day).
- Each meal and snack should contain some quality complex carbohydrate, lean protein and some fat (preferably unsaturated).
- *Be patient!* You didn't gain the weight overnight and it isn't going to come off overnight. A maximum loss of 1–2 pounds per week is healthy if you want to have long-term success.
- Keep a food diary and really analyse it or get some help with making dietary changes.
- Give yourself one cheat day a week and enjoy a special treat. Try to eat well 80–90 per cent of the time and give yourself a break the other 10–20 per cent. You'll find that over time you won't get as much enjoyment from cheating.

Linda has found the secret to her success:

> It seems that if I religiously walk/stretch, watch my diet, take time for myself (I now go to a gym), I have gone from 200 pounds [14 st 4] to 180 pounds [12 st 12]. My symptoms seem much better as long as I follow my schedule, which I am happy with, although I've come to accept that some days my symptoms will come and go, but nothing like it used to be! I still read anything I can get my hands on about thyroid and receive Mary Shomon's thyroid newsletter every month to keep up with new research. No matter what *any* doctors tell me, I trust in myself and how I feel, and do my own research, then I go to the doctors and tell them I want to try something new!

Phyllis is 60 years old, 5 feet tall and weighs a comfortable 114 pounds (8 st 2). She exercises five to six times a week. She says that once she got in touch with the emotional reasons that she ate, she was much more conscious about everything. For 2 years she has maintained her weight on a low-calorie food plan she devised herself that emphasizes lean proteins and vegetables:

I feel great at this weight. I have also been told I look great.
This motivates me to keep watching what I eat. I am now
down to a size 8 and am consistently happy. I might also add,
I do fine when I go out to eat. Whether lunch or dinner, I
maintain by eating a chicken salad. When I go to McDonald's
I select a chicken salad, and I even am able to have an ice-
cream cone. This combination is very satisfying and I look at
it as a treat.

Anna lost 37 pounds when she became hyperthyroid but gained it back,
plus some, under treatment:

They gave me radiation and then I quit smoking and got fat,
gaining more than 50 pounds. My doctor said no diet would
help me. I have tried all the wrong things. Till I tried your
book. I want to thank you for giving me hope and I feel so
good about myself again. I have lost 19 pounds in 75 days –
dropped a few sizes already – and I have to thank you.

Marie went from 185 to 154 pounds (13 st 3 to 11 st) and is still dropping
more:

I used to be a size 20 and am 5 feet tall. I now weigh 11
stone and can wear clothes that I couldn't wear before, and
everyone including neighbours are asking me why I look so
good!

Roberta read about and started following my approach to weight loss for
thyroid patients six months ago:

After reading your diet guide, I was amazed with the
information that my doctors had not told me regarding
hypothyroidism. I wanted to let you know that since I started
taking your advice that is mentioned in your book, I have lost
35 pounds.

On other diets, Barb would lose 5 pounds, then hit a permanent plateau:

> On the diet you recommend, I've lost 12 pounds in 3 months.
> I lost a pound a week for the first 9 pounds and then have
> slowed down to a pound every 2 weeks or so. I'm 5'3" and
> weighed 138 [9 st 12] when I started the diet. I plan to
> follow the outlines of your diet for the rest of my life.

So keep the faith. Keep following my own weight-loss story and stay up on the latest thyroid and weight-loss news at my site: http://www.goodmetabolism.com.

I predict that someday soon you'll be sending me your success story! You can write to me at mshomon@thyroid-info.com, or by mail at:

Mary Shomon
PO Box 565
Kensington
Maryland 20895-0565
USA

Appendices

Appendices

Resources

Updated web links for information on how to buy the various books and products and how to contact the experts mentioned in this book are all featured online at this book's website: http://www.goodmetabolism.com.

At goodmetabolism.com you can also sign up for our e-mail newsletter, *A Weight Off My Mind*, which already has more than 30,000 subscribers. It reports on the latest news on weight-loss nutrition, metabolism, thyroid disease and autoimmune conditions.

MARY SHOMON'S INFORMATION
Thyroid Information

Mary Shomon's Thyroid-Info Website
http://www.thyroid-info.com

A comprehensive site featuring news articles, interviews and information on all facets of thyroid disease, including both conventional and alternative approaches to diagnosis and treatment. Not sponsored by any pharmaceutical companies, so you get thousands of pages of unbiased, patient-orientated information from a leading thyroid patient advocate. Find chats, support groups, online forums and more to help you in your effort to live well with thyroid disease.

Thyroid Top Doctors Directory
http://www.thyroid-info.com/topdrs

A directory of patient-recommended top thyroid practitioners from around the world, organized by country.

Thyroid Site at About.com
http://thyroid.about.com
Founded and managed by Mary Shomon, the Thyroid Site at About.com features hundreds of links to top sites on the net, a weekly newsletter, support community and more.

Living Well with Hypothyroidism: What Your Doctor Doesn't Tell You ...
That You Need to Know (Mary J. Shomon, HarperCollins/Avon, 1st
edition: 2000, 2nd edition: 2005)
http://www.thyroid-info.com/book.htm
A best seller, the 2000 edition of this book went to 20 printings before a revised and updated edition was published in 2005. It has been an Amazon.com Top 40 Health Books Best-seller since 2000 and frequently is on the Amazon Top 100 Best-sellers list. The first in-the-trenches manual about hypothyroidism, the book is written by a patient and offers practical help on every facet of hypothyroidism. Covers alternative medicine approaches, conquering depression, overcoming infertility, having a healthy pregnancy, effective weight loss and even special chapters on hypothyroidism in infants and children, and hypothyroidism after thyroid cancer surgery. The book also offers a comprehensive Resource Guide featuring hundreds of books, websites, organizations, support groups and people who can help you live well. The *Los Angeles Times* has called it a 'first-rate book' that 'challenges patients and their doctors to look deeper and try harder to resolve the complicated symptoms of hypothyroidism'. Available at bookshops and online.

Sticking Out Our Necks Print Newsletter
http://www.thyroid-info.com/subscribe.htm
A bi-monthly 12-page print newsletter posted directly to you that features key thyroid-related conventional and alternative information in an unbiased, patient-orientated format. Order online, or write:

Sticking Out Our Necks/Thyroid-Info
PO Box 656
Kensington, Maryland 20895-0565
USA

Sticking Out Our Necks E-mail Newsletter
http://www.thyroid-info.com/newsletters.htm

A monthly e-mail newsletter featuring key thyroid-related news, developments, links, interviews and more. To subscribe, visit the website or e-mail thyroidnews@thyroid-info.com.

Thyroid Guide to Fertility, Pregnancy and Breastfeeding Success
http://www.thyroid-info.com/pregnancyguide.htm

A 40-page guide that covers the critical relationship between the thyroid gland and nearly every aspect of childbearing. Reviews how undiagnosed thyroid problems can cause infertility or recurrent miscarriage, making it difficult or impossible to get or stay pregnant. Covers thyroid problems and how they can complicate pregnancy, worsen pregnancy symptoms such as morning sickness, fatigue, hair loss and depression, and increase the risk of miscarriage, intrauterine growth retardation, pre-term labour, stillbirth and cognitive problems/mental retardation. Also discusses postpartum thyroid problems and breast-feeding difficulties with thyroid disease, as well as solutions. Order online, or write:

Sticking Out Our Necks/Thyroid-Info
PO Box 565
Kensington, Maryland 20895-0565
USA

Weight-Loss Information

A Weight Off My Mind Newsletter
http://www.thyroid-info.com/dietnews/index.htm

A monthly e-mail newsletter featuring key thyroid-related news, developments, links, interviews and more. To subscribe, visit the website or e-mail diet@thyroidinfo.com.

Autoimmune Disease Information

Living Well with Autoimmune Disease: What Your Doctor Doesn't Tell You ... That You Need to Know (Mary J. Shomon, HarperCollins, 2002)
http://www.autoimmunebook.com

After numerous printings, *Living Well with Autoimmune Disease* has established itself as the definitive guide to understanding mysterious and often difficult-to-pinpoint autoimmune disorders like thyroid disease, Hashimoto's thyroiditis, Graves' disease, multiple sclerosis, rheumatoid arthritis, Sjogren's syndrome, lupus, alopecia, irritable bowel syndrome, psoriasis, Raynaud's and many others. The book offers a roadmap to finding both conventional and alternative diagnosis, treatment, recovery and, in some cases, even prevention or cure! *Alternative Medicine Magazine* has said, '*Living Well with Autoimmune Disease* should not only prove inspirational for those afflicted with these mysterious conditions, but also offers solid, practical advice for getting your health back on track.' Available at bookshops or online.

Autoimmune Report E-mail Newsletter
http://www.thyroid-info.com/autoimmune/news.htm
A monthly e-mail newsletter that reviews the latest conventional and alternative medical journals to bring you breaking information on treatments, including new drugs, diet and supplements and other findings related to autoimmune disease. Subscribe online or via e-mail: autoimmune@thyroid-info.com.

OTHER THYROID AND AUTOIMMUNE DISEASE INFORMATION
Books

Graves' Disease: A Practical Guide (Elaine Moore and Lisa Moore, MacFarland & Company, 2001)
Excellent, comprehensive and well-researched overview of Graves' disease that offers conventional and alternative information on diagnosis and treatment.

Solved: The Riddle of Illness (Stephen E. Langer and James F. Scheer, McGraw Hill – NTC, 3rd edition, 2000)
Highlights the authors' tremendous knowledge of nutritional medicine and the relationship between thyroid disease and many conditions, such as arthritis, obesity, depression, diabetes, heart disease, cancer, sexual problems and much more.

Thyroid Power: Ten Steps to Total Health (Richard Shames and Karilee Halo Shames, Harper Resource, 2001)

Puts some basics of hypothyroidism causes, tests, diagnosis and treatment into a 10-step programme of information that can help patients get properly diagnosed and treated.

Overcoming Thyroid Disorders (David Brownstein, Medical Alternatives Press, 2002)

Good information on holistic and hormonal approaches to thyroid treatment.

Organizations

British Thyroid Foundation (BTF)

PO Box 97, Clifford, Wetherby, West Yorkshire LS23 6XD
http://www.btf-thyroid.org
Affiliated to the doctors' British Thyroid Association. Produces a useful newsletter and simple leaflets covering a wide range of thyroid problems.

Thyroid UK

32 Darcy Road, St Osyth, Clacton-on-Sea, Essex CO16 8QF
http://www.thyroiduk.org
webenquiries@thyroiduk.org
Produces a thought-provoking newsletter and information pack. Useful source of information about animal thyroid preparations, and the potential links between thyroid problems, myalgic encephalomyelitis (ME, or chronic fatigue syndrome, CFS) and adrenal failure. Maintains a list of doctors interested in an alternative approach to thyroid problems.

Thyroid Eye Disease Association

Solstice, Sea Road, Winchelsea Beach, East Sussex TN36 4LH
tedassn@eclipse.co.uk
Useful newsletter and leaflets specifically for people with thyroid eye disease. Associated with British Thyroid Association and founder member of Thyroid Federation International.

Changing Faces

The Squire Centre, 33–37 University Street, London WC1E 6JN
http://www.changingfaces.org.uk
info@changingfaces.org.uk
Charity dedicating to helping people manage their altered appearance more successfully. Practical advice and support for rebuilding self-confidence.

Institute for Complementary Medicine (ICM)

PO Box 194, London SE16 7QZ
www.i-c-m.org.uk
info@i-c-m.org.uk

British Complementary Medicine Association

PO Box 5122, Bournemouth BH8 0WG
http://www.bcma.co.uk
info@bcma.co.uk

Thyroid Federation International

797 Princess Street, Suite 304, Kingston, Ontario K7L 1G1
http://www.thyroid-fed.org
tfi@on.aibn.com
Useful information on thyroid problems and links to other organizations worldwide. Good source of information on how to start a thyroid patients' group.

Thyroid Foundation of America

410 Stuart Street, Boston, MA 02116
[+001] 617-534-1500
http://www.allthyroid.org
The main US organization involved in thyroid education and outreach.

American Autoimmune Related Diseases Association

22100 Gratiot Avenue, East Detroit, MI 48021

[+001] 810-776-3900

http://www.aarda.org/

aarda@aol.com

Information about more than 50 different autoimmune disorders, including Hashimoto's disease and Graves' disease. This website and organization provide general information about autoimmune disorders and profiles of specific diseases.

The Endocrine Society

8401 Connecticut Avenue, Suite 900, Chevy Chase, MD 20815-5817

[+001] 301-941-0200 Fax: [+001] 301-941-0259

http://www.endo-society.org

endostaff@endo-society.org

A group with a mission to promote the understanding of hormones and endocrinology and the impact of this knowledge on preventing, diagnosing and treating disease, including thyroid disease and obesity. The group publishes a number of journals and maintains an informational website.

Medical Journal

Journal of Clinical Endocrinology and Metabolism

The Endocrine Society, 8401 Connecticut Avenue, Suite 900, Chevy Chase, MD 20815

[+001] 301-941-0200

http://jcem.endojournals.org

The medical journal that focuses on the cross-section between thyroid disease and weight loss.

TESTING LABORATORIES

Individual Wellbeing Diagnostic Laboratory (IWDL)

Parkgate House, 356 West Barnes Lane, New Malden, Surrey KT3 6NB

http://www.iwdl.net

Yorktest Laboratories Ltd
Murton Way, Osbaldwick, York YO19 5US
http://www.allergy-testing.com

ONLINE DIET SERVICES AND TOOLS

Ediets Online – Recommended Site
http://www.ediets.com/
At Ediets, members fill out a diet profile, then choose from a variety of diets such as Atkins, the Zone and Jenny Craig. With a personalized programme that includes daily meal plans, workout programmes and shopping lists, members enter information into the system to track progress.

Physique Transformation – Recommended Site
http://www.physiquetransformation.com
Ric Rooney and Bart Hanks of Physique Transformation provide a Personal Food Analyst software programme that analyses your diet and generates a personalized plan for reaching weight-loss goals.

Weight Watchers – Recommended Site
http://www.weightwatchers.com
Members of Weight Watchers sign up and are allocated a certain number of daily points. Members keep track of points using interactive journals, trackers and calculators and can join online or in local communities for support.

DietPower – Recommended Site
http://www.dietpower.com
DietPower is weight and nutrition management software that helps you set weight-loss goals based on your personal information, diet and fitness level. Record your exercise and meals using the extensive food database to track your calories and any nutrients you might be missing. DietPower is available for a free 15-day trial.

Calorie King
http://www.calorieking.com

Founded by Allan Borushek, a clinical dietician, the Calorie King offers an online weight-management programme that includes recommended meal plans, exercise routines and help in choosing fitness goals. The site also includes recipes, calculators, fitness and health articles, forums, chat rooms and more.

FitDay
http://www.fitday.com

FitDay is an online tracking system that offers a personal journal to track the foods you eat and daily activities. FitDay analyses your diet and exercise and offers reports on calories, nutrients, weight loss and more. A subscription is free.

FitWatch
http://www.fitwatch.com

FitWatch offers a comprehensive online tracking system for nutrition and exercise. Members can enter meals and exercise activities into journals using online databases.

MyBodyComp.com
http://www.mybodycomp.com/

This website offers an online body fat monitor designed to help you track body fat percentage, lean body mass, waist-to-hip ratio, calories burned and more. Subscription is free.

Nutritional Analysis Tool
http://www.ag.uiuc.edu/food-lab/nat/

This online nutritional analysis tool allows users to analyse foods and meals for a variety of nutrients. The programme is free.

Health Central Cool Tools
http://www.healthcentral.com/cooltools/ct_fitness/ct_fitness.cfm

Health Central offers free fitness and weight-loss tools including a body mass index calculator, fitness profile, healthy weight calculator and fat test.

WEIGHT-LOSS INFORMATION WEBSITES
General Sites

Weight Watchers

Millennium House, Ludlow Road, Maidenhead, Berkshire SL6 2SL

http://www.weightwatchers.co.uk

Weight Watchers offers local programmes and meetings, or Weight Watchers Online. Members can search the website for meeting locations where they receive the Winning Points Plan – a diet system in which members are allocated daily points depending on their weight and goals. Online weight-loss services include Weight Watchers Etools and Weight Watchers Online, which includes a journal, a weight tracker, meal plans, point calculators, a recipe search and more.

Overeaters Anonymous

PO Box 19, Stretford, Manchester, M32 9EB

http://www.oagb.org.uk

A recovery programme using the Twelve Steps to help members recover from overeating.

WebMD

http://my.webmd.com/health_and_wellness/food_nutrition

Excellent, comprehensive information, news and resources for weight-loss support.

iVillage Fitness

http://www.ivillage.com/topics/fitness/0,,165513,00.html

iVillage offers articles, tips and information on weight loss including diet programmes, eating habits, exercise, trends, strength-training and more.

MEDLINEPlus – Weight Loss/Dieting

http://www.nlm.nih.gov/medlineplus/weightlossdieting.html

This website run by the US National Institutes of Health posts basic information and the latest news in weight loss, nutrition and science.

Weight Loss at About.com
http://weightloss.about.com
Extensive database of articles and resources on weight loss, including well-known diets like Atkins and Weight Watchers, info on the latest diet trends, and weight-loss options and tips on creating a healthy lifestyle.

Support Groups Online

Thyroid Diet Support Group
http://www.goodmetabolism
Join other thyroid dieters at the forum specifically for *The Thyroid Diet* and for discussion of how to lose weight despite thyroid disease.

About Weight Loss Forum
http://forums.about.com/ab-weightloss/start/
The About Weight Loss Forum offers support if you're trying to lose weight. Register for free, and post questions or search through the forum for specific information about diets, nutrition, diet buddies, obesity and other popular topics.

Real Losers
http://www.real-losers.com/
This website offers plenty of support for people who want to lose weight. You'll find success stories, informational articles to help educate and inspire you and an extensive support network including chats, forum boards and buddy systems.

3 Fat Chicks Community Weight Loss Journal
http://3fatchicks.com/journals/weblog
One way to stay on track is to keep a weight-loss journal. 3fatchicks.com offers an online community journal to help you stay motivated. The public aspect holds you accountable for your weight loss, and you'll find lots of support from other members.

Diettalk.com
http://www.diettalk.com
Diettalk offers free support through their forums, which include general support, support for specific diets and programmes, emergency support and more. Their site also offers chats, articles and a free newsletter.

My Diet Buddy
http://www.mydietbuddy.com
Mydietbuddy.com matches members with one another according to lifestyle and diet/fitness goals.

Low-Fat, Low-Carb, Low-Glycaemic, Healthy Recipes

Glycaemic Index
http://diabetes.about.com/library/mendosagi/ngilists.htm
Rick Mendosa provides a comprehensive table of foods categorized by glycaemic index (GI) and glycaemic load values, along with basic information about what GI means and how to use the table.

iVillage Low-Fat Diet Plan Info
http://www.ivillage.com/topics/fitness/0,,415981,00.html
This website provides a starting point for basic information on a variety of low-fat diets including Weight Watchers, Jenny Craig, Nutri/System and more. The site offers essential information, articles, message boards, newsletters, tools and recipes.

Low-fat Recipes from 3 Fat Chicks
http://www.3fatchicks.com/cookbook/
This website lists over 800 low-fat recipes that include calories, protein, fibre, fat gram, sodium, carbohydrates and Weight Watcher points. Recipes are divided into categories and are free.

Low-fat Cooking
http://lowfatcooking.about.com/
Hundreds of low-fat recipes for breakfast, lunch, dinner and more. Also offers articles, eating tips, meal planners and facts about low-fat eating.

AICR – Recipe Corner
http://www.aicr.org/information/recipe/index.lasso
The American Institute for Cancer Research offers free healthy recipes for
soups, salads, entrées, veggies, desserts and more.

WEIGHT-LOSS BOOKS, COOKBOOKS
Diet and Weight-Loss Books

Atkins Diet
http://atkins.com/
The Atkins home page provides information about the Atkins diet, including how it works, food and recipes, motivation and success stories. You can
sign up for a free Atkins account to keep a food journal, shopping list,
recipe box and more.

Zone Diet
http://www.zoneperfect.com/Site/Content/index.asp
The Zone online magazine provides support for those following the Zone
diet. The website provides an online cookbook, success stories, meal plans,
fitness calculators and more.

Blood Type Diet/Eat Right 4 Your Type
http://www.dadamo.com/
This website provides information and education about the Blood Type
diet. The site includes a health library, recipe database, columns and articles about diet and health.

No-Grain Diet
http://www.mercola.com/nograindiet/
The website provides information and support for dieters. It includes
expert information, success stories, newsletters and more.

South Beach Diet
http://www.southbeachdiet.com
This interactive website offers support for those on the South Beach diet. Sign up for daily tips, recipes and guidance from the author, Dr Agatston, and use interactive tools to track weight and meals and generate shopping lists.

Sugar Busters
http://www.sugarbusters.com
This website covers the basics of the Sugar Busters diet. Get information about how to follow the diet and sign on to the message board for information and support.

Fat Flush Diet
http://www.fatflush.com/
Anne Louise Gittleman's website provides articles and information about the Fat Flush diet. The site also includes support boards, product information and other dieting resources.

8 Minutes in the Morning
http://www.jorgecruise.com/
The Jorge Cruise website provides a starting place for those interested in the programme 8 Minutes in the Morning. The site offers free coaching, success stories, newsletters, support and product information.

Body for Life
http://www.bodyforlife.com/
The Body for Life website provides basic information about the programme, including free downloadable strength-training programmes. The site also includes bulletin boards, articles and chat capabilities.

Protein Power
http://www.eatprotein.com/
The Protein Power website offers information about the Protein Power Lifeplan, including books, recipes and articles. Also includes fitness products, community support and chat capabilities.

Carbohydrate Addict's Diet
http://www.carbohydrateaddicts.com/
This website offers a list of books, articles, quizzes and success stories relating to the Carbohydrate Addict's diet.

Metabolic Typing Diet
http://www.metabolictypingdiet.com/index2.html
This website discusses the Metabolic Typing diet and includes interactive quizzes for discovering your metabolic type, choosing foods, as well as providing other information about the diet.

Schwarzbein Principle
http://www.schwarzbeinprinciple.com/
The Schwarzbein Principle website offers basic information about the diet including nutrition, stress-management, toxins, exercise and hormones. The site also includes articles about supplements, health news and more.

Ultimate Weight Solution: The 7 Keys of Weight Loss Freedom (Phillip McGraw, Free Press, 2003)
Dr Phil focuses on taking readers through a weight-loss plan based on the emotional reasons people overeat. Readers will learn how to make a weight-loss plan, receive tools to plan meals and learn how to avoid emotional eating.

Fat and Furious (Loree Taylor Jordan, L.T.J. Associates, 2004)
A look at weight-loss issues from the mind–body perspective and also including thyroid-related information.

Fat Tracker (Karen Xhisholm, Fat Tracker Publications, 2003)
http://www.thefattracker.com
Tracking guide to keep track of whichever diet you follow, including water, nutrients, exercise and more.

Best Cookbooks for Weight Loss

Prevention's Stop Dieting & Lose Weight Cookbook (Mary Jo Platt, Rodale Press, 1998)

The book details easy ways to lose weight by reducing fats, eating healthy foods and making exercise a priority. Skipping the latest miracle diet, the more than 275 recipes are low in fat and calories.

American Heart Association Meals in Minutes Cookbook (American Heart Association, Times Books, 2000)

This cookbook provides over 200 heart-healthy meals that can be prepared in minutes. The emphasis is on easy meals that can be put together in 20 minutes or less.

Splendid Low-Carbing, Splendid Low-Carbing for Life and More Splendid Low-Carbing (Jennifer Eloff)

http://www.sweety.com

A wonderful selection of low-carb recipes, including terrific desserts.

The Low-Carb Comfort Food Cookbook (Michael R. Eades, John Wiley & Sons, 2002)

This book offers over 300 low-carb recipes for comfort foods such as pancakes, ice cream, cookies and pasta. Also provides cooking tips and articles about weight loss and cravings.

Dr Atkins' Quick and Easy New Diet Cookbook (Robert C. Atkins, Fireside, 1997)

If you're following the Atkins diet, this book offers quick and easy recipes that are very low in carbs and high in protein and fat.

Weight Watchers New Complete Cookbook (Weight Watchers International Inc. Staff, John Wiley & Sons, 1998)

This cookbook is designed for the Weight Watcher's programme and provides 500 recipes, each of which is assigned food points based on fat, fibre and calories. Recipes are varied and cover sauces, breads, meat, vegetarian dishes, pasta and more.

Stop the Clock! Cooking (Cheryl Forberg, Penguin Putnam, 2003)
Chef and registered dietician Cheryl Forberg offers over 100 healthy recipes that focus on anti-ageing ingredients such as berries, fish, tomatoes, soy, grains and more.

The Good Carb Cookbook: Secrets of Eating Low on the Glycemic Index (Sandra Woodruff, Avery Penguin Putnam, 2001)
Sandra Woodruff explains carbs and which foods affect blood sugar and cravings. Low-carb, low-calorie recipes cover all types of meals.

Stella's Kitchen: Creative Cooking for Fun, Flavour and a Lean, Strong Body (Estella Juarez, On Target Publications, 2003)
Estella Juarez provides a variety of recipes targeted to exercise and fitness enthusiasts. She discusses the basics of choosing ingredients and provides tips on cooking.

The Vegetarian Gourmet's Easy Low-Fat Favourites (Bobbie Hinman, Surrey Books, 2002)
This cookbook provides over 300 low-fat, vegetarian recipes using fresh fruits and vegetables, whole grains and beans. Nutritional breakdown is included as well as suggested menus.

DIET FOODS

Iherb
http://www.iherb.com
An excellent website for a variety of diet foods, low-carb products and supplements.

Carbolite
http://www.carbolitedirect.com/
This website offers low-carb, sugar-free diet foods in bulk or combo specials.

Grains & Greens
http://www.grainsandgreens.com/merchant.ihtml
This online food shop offers Atkins diet products and a variety of natural foods, beverages, appliances and more.

Synergy Diet
http://www.synergydiet.com/?AID=8110879&PID=1173325
Synergy Diet is an online shop offering a large selection of low-carbohydrate, sugar-free, high-protein foods, beverages and supplements.

HERBS/SUPPLEMENT INFORMATION

Iherb
http://www.iherb.com
Online retailer features reliable information about supplements. A source for most of the supplements discussed here.

Consumer Lab
http://www.consumerlab.com/
This site is a great resource for people interested in taking herbal supplements. ConsumerLab.com offers independent testing of popular herbs to help consumers evaluate the safety of vitamins, minerals, herbal products and more.

CraniYums Supplements
http://www.craniyums.com/
Serotonin- and dopamine-balancing supplements for weight loss.

Drug Digest
http://www.drugdigest.org/DD/DVH/Herbs
This comprehensive site provides detailed information about drugs, herbs and supplements. Also includes interactions with medications and information about specific conditions.

FDA – Overview of Dietary Supplements
http://vm.cfsan.fda.gov/~dms/ds-oview.html
This article offers basic information about what dietary supplements are, how to read labels and more.

WebMD Drugs and Supplements
http://my.webmd.com/medical_information/drug_and_herb/default.htm
This section of WebMD provides a searchable database containing information about a variety of drugs, herbs and supplements. Also includes articles about dietary supplements and their use and effectiveness.

WEIGHT-LOSS DRUG INFORMATION

About Weight Loss – Products & Supplements
http://weightloss.about.com/cs/products/
This list of links provides information about popular weight-loss pills and products.

Diet Pills
http://www.diet-i.com/diet-pills.htm
This article offers in-depth information about diet pills, both prescription and over the counter. Describes popular diet drugs, side-effects, pros and cons.

iVillage – Weight Loss Drugs & Surgery
http://www.ivillage.com/topics/fitness/0,10707,192161,00.html
In this section of iVillage, users will find information and articles about different weight-loss drugs and their safety and effectiveness.

Obesity Meds & Research
http://www.obesity-news.com/newdrugs.htm
This page details information about weight-loss drugs in use, in development, and those that are available over the counter.

Medscape Drug Info
http://www.medscape.com/druginfo/

Mesotherapy

Dr Lionel Bissoon, DO
[+001] 212-579-9136
http://mesoestetik.com/home.html
http://www.mesotherapy.com

FITNESS/EXERCISE INFORMATION

Exercise at About.com
http://exercise.about.com
This site provides comprehensive information about all aspects of exercise including cardio, strength-training, apparel, gear and more. Includes exercise articles, support forum, newsletter, free workouts and product reviews.

ExRx Exercise Information
http://www.exrx.net/ExInfo.html
ExRx is an excellent website offering basic information about getting started with exercise. Articles cover fitness components, injury prevention, motor development and more.

Fitness Online
http://www.fitnessonline.com/
Fitness Online contains a variety of information about fitness and exercise including getting fit, eating healthy, building muscle and losing weight. Includes online calculators, expert advice and instructional workouts.

IDEAfit.com
http://www.ideafit.com/
The IDEA Health and Fitness Association provides health and fitness news as well as workout articles and fitness facts covering all aspects of exercise for fitness enthusiasts.

Internet Fitness
http://www.internetfitness.com/
Internet Fitness provides information about exercise, walking, running, motivation, strength-training, home fitness and more. An authority in his or her field moderates each category.

Just Move
http://www.justmove.org/home.cfm
This site run by the American Heart Association offers news and information relating to fitness, health and weight loss. It provides an online forum and fitness diary to track your workouts.

Workout.com
http://www.workout.com
Workout.com offers a library of professionally developed exercise programmes, exercise instructions, video demonstrations, community support and more. Workouts are categorized according to goals such as muscle development, cardiovascular conditioning and weight loss.

MEDLINE Plus – Exercise/Physical Fitness
http://www.nlm.nih.gov/medlineplus/exercisephysicalfitness.html
MEDLINE offers general fitness information that includes getting started, activity tips and exercise for children and seniors. Also provides the latest news on physical activity and links to other helpful resources.

Jim Karas' Exercise Instruction
http://www.jimkaras.com/instruction.cfm
Run by personal trainer Jim Karas, this website provides instructions for a variety of exercises using equipment such as resistance bands, dumbbells and exercise balls. The site also includes exercise logs, fitness articles and a community forum for support.

Popular Fitness Exercise Instruction
http://www.popularfitness.com/exercise/index.shtml
This website's exercise instruction page offers video demonstrations for basic exercises for major muscle groups. The site also provides exercise and fitness articles and workout programmes.

Fitness Books

Body for Life (Bill Phillips and Michael D'Orso, HarperCollins, 1999)
This book explains the 12-week programme, including strength-training workouts, cardio, nutrition and supplements. Includes blank logs to keep track of exercise and diet.

Strength Training for Dummies (Suzanne Schlosberg and Liz Neporent, For Dummies, 2000)
Fitness professionals discuss the basics of weight-training in simple terms, providing readers with a step-by-step process for setting up a strength-training programme. Chapters cover types of equipment, tips on technique and illustrations of basic exercises.

Smart Exercise (Covert Bailey, Mariner Books, 1996)
Bailey does a nice job of explaining the basic concepts of fitness and weight loss. He explains physiology in simple terms and describes how the body builds muscles, burns fat and more.

Getting Stronger (Bill Pearl, Shelter Publications, 2001)
This well-written book covers all aspects of weight-training for beginners and body-builders alike. It includes sport-specific training for a variety of sports along with detailed instructions and pictures.

Stretching (Bob Anderson, Shelter Publications, 2001)
This excellent book explains the basics of stretching, then provides an extensive list of stretches (including pictures) for the entire body. There's a section on stretching for specific sports and information on specific conditions such as back pain.

Getting in Shape (Bob Anderson, Ed Burke and Bill Pearl, Shelter Publications, 1994)
This illustrated book provides basic workouts for men and women. The authors discuss the basic components of fitness, offer programmes for work, travel and the gym and move into discussions about food, health, pregnancy and more.

Fitness for Dummies (Suzanne Schlosberg and Liz Neporent, For Dummies, 1999)

This book for beginners helps readers plan a well-rounded fitness programme by explaining the basics of exercise without any confusing jargon. Topics cover cardio, weight-training, basic nutrition, supplements, myths and more.

Top Fitness/Exercise Videos for Beginners

Winsor Pilates
http://www.winsorpilates.com

A programme that features a set of various videos for doing mat Pilates at home. Videos offer a variety of routines to help tone and sculpt the entire body.

Pilates for Dummies (2001)

This 60-minute workout is perfect for beginners, explaining the fundamentals of Pilates training. The workout includes basic movements and goes at a slow pace.

Yoga Journal's Yoga for Beginners (Patricia Walden, 1990)

For beginners, this is the most comprehensive video about yoga available. The instructor leads exercisers through a basic yoga workout, emphasizing form and posture through the 60-minute routine.

Kathy Smith's Step Workout (Kathy Smith, 2001)

This is the perfect starting point for beginning steppers. Kathy Smith provides three progressively more difficult step segments, and exercisers move through the segments as they become conditioned.

Fat Burning for Dummies with Gay Gasper (2001)

This easy-to-follow routine introduces 10 basic aerobic moves, allowing beginner exercisers to learn the fundamentals of cardio exercise. The video shows on-screen modifications and includes safety tips.

15-Minute Workouts for Dummies (Gay Gasper, 2003)

Gay Gasper's newest video offers four workouts, each one focused on a different muscle group: thighs, arms, legs and abs. The workout has on-screen modifications, tips and safety suggestions.

FIRM Basics Series (Fat Burning, Abs, Buns and Thighs, Sculpting with Weights), 1986

The FIRM offers an excellent series of videos introducing new exercisers to strength-training. Instructors offer tips on proper form and provide brief aerobic sections in between weight work.

Ease into Fitness (Karen Voight, 1999)

Karen Voight offers a very basic, low-impact workout for new exercisers and seniors using a resistance band. The exercises are easy to understand, and Karen provides excellent instruction.

Beginner's Stretch for Flexibility (Tamilee Webb, 2000)

Tamilee Webb provides a basic 30-minute flexibility workout. This relaxing routine involves traditional stretches along with easy yoga poses for a nice introduction to stretching.

Leslie Sansone's In-Home Walk (Leslie Sansone, 2000)

This easy-to-follow video offers a 2-mile walking workout that can be done in the home. Perfect for beginners.

Yoga Stress Relief for Beginners (Suzanne Deason, 1998)

This 17-minute video offers a relaxing series of poses to introduce new exercisers to yoga.

OTHER PRODUCTS OF INTEREST

Belleruth Naparstek's Weight-Loss Guided Visualization Audio/CD

This guided weight-loss CD uses imagery to help users heighten serotonin levels to reduce appetite and to convert fat into focused energy and muscle. The 60-minute audio also helps listeners learn to appreciate their bodies.

**Light Boxes for Light Treatment/Seasonal Affective Disorder Therapy
(Sunbox Company)**
http://www.sunbox.com
Excellent quality, selection and service, offering the nation's largest selection of various lamps specifically designed for light treatment. Also features articles and information on light therapy.

Dr Levine's Ultimate Weight-Loss Formula™
http://www.thindoctor.com
There are 17 grams of fibre per serving. The formula comes in chocolate, vanilla cream, orange cream, hazelnut and raspberry.

EXPERTS

The following practitioners and experts provided information or ideas as I developed this book.

David Brownstein, MD
David Brownstein is a board-certified family doctor and practitioner of holistic medicine. He is the medical director of the Center for Holistic Medicine in West Bloomfield, Michigan. Dr Brownstein specializes in the use of vitamins, minerals, herbs and natural hormones. He is the author of three popular books: *The Miracle of Natural Hormones*, *Overcoming Thyroid Disorders* and *Overcoming Arthritis*. His website is located at http://www.drbrownstein.com. He can be reached at 4173 Fieldbrook, West Bloomfield, MI 48323; [+001] 248-851-3372 or [+001] 888-647-5616; info@drbrownstein.com.

Hyla Cass, MD
Hyla Cass is an integrative and holistic physician and psychiatrist, with expertise in natural treatments for stress, anxiety, depression, nutritional and hormonal imbalances. She is the best-selling author of a number of books, including *Natural Highs*. Her website is located at http://www.cassmd.com and she can be reached by e-mail at hyla@cassmd.com.

Udo Erasmus, PhD

Udo Erasmus is a nutritionist and researcher who has spent more than 15 years exploring the practical aspects of fats. He pioneered technology for pressing and packaging fresh oils and created the well-known Udo's Oils series of essential fatty acid products. He is also author of the best-selling book *Fats That Heal, Fats That Kill*. His website is located at http://www.udoerasmus, and he offers private consultations by phone from his office in Canada. He can be reached at admin@udoerasmus.com.

Bruce Fife, ND

Bruce Fife is a certified nutritionist and naturopathic physician. He is the author of several books including *The Healing Miracles of Coconut Oil* and *Eat Fat, Look Thin*. He can be reached at PO Box 25203, Colorado Springs, CO 80936 or thyroidhealth@adelphia.net.

Ted Friedman, MD

Ted Friedman is an associate professor of medicine at UCLA's endocrinology division and an endocrinologist in private practice. His website is located at http://www.goodhormonehealth.com. Dr Friedman's practice is located at 8737 Beverly Boulevard, Suite 203, Los Angeles, CA 90048. For more information, ring [+001] 310-335-0327, or e-mail appointments@goodhormonehealth.com.

Ann Louise Gittleman, PhD

Ann Louise Gittleman is author of a number of best-selling books on nutrition and hormones, including *Before the Change* and *The Fat Flush Plan*. She has worked in both the public and private health sectors with thousands of clients. Her website and contact information is located at http://www.fatflush.com.

Donna Hurlock, MD

Donna Hurlock is an Alexandria, Virginia-based gynaecologist and a certified menopause clinician. She also has a special interest in wellness, disease prevention, nutrition and treating hypothyroidism via alternative medicine approaches. Her website is located at http://www.dhurlock.yourmd.com. She can be reached at 205 S. Whiting Street, Suite 303, Alexandria, VA 22304; tel [+001] 703-823-1533.

Dave Junno PsyD

Dave Junno is a psychologist, coach and author of *Lowering High Cholesterol and Reducing Your Risk of Heart Disease – Ready or Not!* E-mail him at drjunno@drjunno.com or visit his website at http://www.lower-high-cholesterol-ready-or-not.com.

Stephen Langer, MD

Stephen Langer is a holistic physician in private practice, with expertise in holistic and integrative therapies, anti-ageing medicine and hormonal, thyroid and nutritional conditions. He is also the author of numerous books, including *Solved: The Riddle of Illness*, which is co-authored with James Scheer. Dr Langer provides in-office and phone consultations regarding thyroiditis, hypothyroidism, fibromyalgia, chronic fatigue, ortho-molecular medicine, optimal nutrition, metabolic medicine and food allergies. He can be reached at 3031 Telegraph Avenue, Suite 230, Berkeley, CA 94705; tel [+001] 510-548-7384.

Scott Levine, MD

Scott Levine is board certified in internal medicine and maintains a practice in Orlando, Florida. He created Dr Levine's Ultimate Weight Loss Formula, a fibre-based weight-loss aid. His website is at http://www.thindoctor.com and he can be reached at 7350 Sandlake Commons Boulevard, Suite 2217, Orlando, FL 32819; tel [+001] 407-354-0001.

Jim McCauley

Since childhood, Jim knew that he wanted to work in the food industry, either as a chef or owning his own restaurant. Before achieving that, he spent 15 years working in the entertainment industry, often helping out friends who owned and managed restaurants. In 1995, Jim moved to New York and enrolled at the French Culinary Institute (FCI). After graduating from FCI, Jim worked at a three-star Hudson Valley restaurant outside of New York City, then took a job as a chef working in corporate dining. Two years ago, Jim was diagnosed with diabetes, so he's turned his training, knowledge and love of food to working on healthier and appropriate recipes that taste great. He can be reached at jim.mccauley@verizon.net.

Joseph Mercola, DO

Joseph Mercola is a Chicago-area osteopathic physician and natural medicine expert who specializes in treating metabolic and immune system disorders. He also runs a popular alternative medicine website at http://www.mercola.com. Mercola is co-author of the best-selling book *The No-Grain Diet*. He can be reached at Optimal Wellness Centre, 1443 W. Schaumburg Road, Schaumburg, IL 60194; tel [+001] 847-985-1777.

Byron Richards, CCN

Byron Richards is a pioneer in the field of clinical nutrition, with over 18 years of experience helping patients recover from serious health issues as well as helping those interested in preventative health. A nutritionist in private practice, he is author of the book *Mastering Leptin*. His website is at http://www.masteringleptin.com.

Marie Savard, MD

Marie Savard is an internationally-known internist and women's health expert, author and patients' rights advocate. She is the founder of the Savard System and author of two books: *How to Save Your Own Life: The Savard System for Managing – and Controlling – Your Health Care* and *The Savard Health Record: A Six-Step System for Managing Your Health Care*. Dr Savard's website is at http://www.drsavard.com. She can be reached at Savard Systems, 54 Churchill Drive, York, PA 17403; tel [+001] 877-728-2737 or [+001] 717-747-0936.

Richard Shames, MD/Karilee Halo Shames RN, PhD

Richard Shames is a holistic physician in private practice and is co-author of a number of health-related books, including *Thyroid Power*. Dr Shames also provides telephone consultations. Karilee Halo Shames is a clinical specialist in psychiatric nursing and a certified holistic nurse with a PhD in holistic studies. She has maintained a private practice in collaboration with Dr Richard Shames for 20 years, specializing in comprehensive treatment aspects of energy-depletion illnesses. She is co-author of *Thyroid Power*. Richard and Karilee Shames can be reached at PO Box 593, Sebastopol, CA 95473-0593; tel [+001] 415-472-2343; their website at http://www.thyroidpower.com; or by e-mail, thyroidpower@aol.com.

Jacob Teitelbaum, MD

Jacob Teitelbaum is board certified in internal medicine. For over a decade he has worked with chronic fatigue syndrome, fibromyalgia and thyroid patients. He has a specialized practice in Annapolis, Maryland and is director of the Annapolis Research Center for Effective FMS/CFS Therapies. He is author of the best-selling book *From Fatigued to Fantastic*. Dr Teitelbaum's website is at http://www.endfatigue.com, and he can be reached at 466 Forelands Road, Annapolis, MD 21401; tel [+001] 410-573-5389.

Silvia Treves

Silvia Treves is a certified personal trainer, specializing in Pilates mat exercise and rehabilitative exercise and strength/flexibility training, working in the Montgomery County and northwest Washington, DC area. Her clients have included Kirk Douglas and a number of other celebrities, and her expertise is working with seniors and people with chronic disease and physical limitations. She can be reached at [+001] 301-654-3976 or silvia-treves50@yahoo.com.

Paige Waehner

Paige Waehner is a fitness and exercise expert and writer and serves as exercise guide at the About.com Exercise site, located at http://exercise.about.com.

Ken Woliner, MD, ABFP

Ken Woliner is a board-certified family physician in private practice in Boca Raton. He can be reached at Holistic Family Medicine, 2499 Glades Road, #106A, Boca Raton, FL 33431; tel [+001] 561-620-7779; knw6@cornell.edu.

Selected References

Abbott Laboratories. *Meridia (sibutramine hydrochloride monohydrate) Product Information.* May 2002.
http://www.rxabbott.com/pdf/meridia.pdf

'Absorption and Transportation of Nutrients', *NutriStrategy* (from National Institutes of Health National Institute of Diabetes and Digestive Kidney Diseases) 2001.
http://www.nutristrategy.com/digestion.htm

Alpor, C. M. 'Effects of Chronic Peanut Consumption on Energy Balance and Hedonics', *International Journal of Obesity* 2002; 26(8): 1129–37

American Journal of Clinical Nutrition, 2002; 75: 476–83

Anoja, S., *et al.* 'Antidiabetic Effects of Panax Ginseng Berry Extract and the Identification of an Effective Component', *Diabetes* 2002; 51: 1851–58

Arnot, Robert. *Dr Bob Arnot's Revolutionary Weight Control Program* (Little, Brown and Company, 1997)

Atkins, Robert C. *Dr Atkins' New Diet Revolution* (Avon Books, 2002)

Backgrounder: Why Sleep Matters, National Sleep Foundation website, http://www.sleepfoundation.org/nsaw/pk_background.html, March 2002

Balsiger, B. M., *et al.* 'Ten and More Years After Vertical Banded Gastroplasty as Primary Operation for Morbid Obesity', *Journal of the American Medical Association* Oct 27, 1999; 282(16): 1530–38

Barclay, Laurie. 'Topiramate Useful for Binge Eating Disorder in Obesity', *American Journal of Psychiatry* February 2003; 160: 255–61

Barkeling, B., *et al.* 'Short-term Effects of Sibutramine (Reductil) on Appetite and Eating Behaviour and the Long-term Therapeutic Outcome', *International Journal of Obesity* June 2003; 27(6): 693–700

Behavior Risk Factor Surveillance System, Trends Data, 2001. Centers for Disease Control and Prevention, National Center for Chronic Disease Prevention and Health Promotion, Division of Adult and Community Health. February 18, 2003. http://www.cdc.gov/brfss/index.htm

Benzphetamine. RXlist.com.
 http://www.rxlist.com/frame/display.cgi?drug=DIDREX.

Blackburn, George L. and Laura C. Bevis. 'The Obesity Epidemic: Prevention and Treatment of the Metabolic Syndrome CME', *Medscape.* http://www.medscape.com/viewprogram/2015_index

Blankson, Henrietta, *et al.* 'Conjugated Linoleic Acid Reduces Body Fat Mass in Overweight and Obese Humans', *Journal of Nutrition* 2000; 130: 2943–48

BMI for Adults, Body Mass Index Formula. Centers for Disease Control and Prevention, National Center for Chronic Disease Prevention and Health Promotion, Division of Nutrition and Physical Activity. April 21, 2003. http://www.cdc.gov/nccdphp/dnpa/bmi/bmi-adult-formula.htm

Body Mass Index (BMI) Table. Centers for Disease Control and Prevention, National Center for Chronic Disease Prevention and Health Promotion, Division of Nutrition and Physical Activity. April 21, 2003. http://www.cdc.gov/nccdphp/dnpa/bmi/00binaries/bmi-adults.pdf

Brain, Marshall. 'How Food Works', *HowStuffWorks.com.*
 http://home.howstuff
works.com/food.htm/printable

Bray, G. A., *et al.* 'A Six-Month Randomized, Placebo Controlled, Dose-Ranging Trial of Topiramate for Weight Loss in Obesity', *Obesity Research* 2003; 11: 722–33

Brownstein, David. *The Miracle of Natural Hormones* (Medical Alternative Press, Inc., 1999)
———. *Overcoming Arthritis* (Medical Alternatives Press, Inc., 2001)
———. *Overcoming Thyroid Disorders* (Medical Alternatives Press, 2002)

Brunova, Jana, *et al.* 'Hyperthyroidism Therapy and Weight Gain', *Abstracts*, 84th annual meeting of the Endocrine Society, June 2002

Bupropion. RXList.com.
 http://www.rxlist.com/frame/display.cgi?drug=Wellbutrin

Cabot, Sandra. *The Liver Cleansing Diet* (SCB International, 1996)

Carney, D. E. and E. D. Tweddell. 'Double Blind Evaluation of Long Acting Diethylpropion Hydrochloride in Obese Patients from a General Practice', *Medical Journal Australia* January 1975; 1(1): 13–15

Cass, Hyla and Patrick Holford. *Natural Highs* (Avery, 2002)

Clinical Guidelines on the Identification, Evaluation and Treatment of Overweight and Obesity in Adults: The Evidence Report. National Institutes of Health; National Heart, Lung and Blood Institute; and National Institute of Diabetes and Digestive and Kidney Diseases. NIH Publication Number 98-4083. September 1998.
http://www.nhlbi.nih.gov/guidelines/obesity/ob_gdlns.htm

Cohen, Sir Philip. *Understanding Insulin Signaling.* July 12, 2000.
http://www.wellcome.ac.uk/en/1/awtpubnwswlkbcksp3inssig.html

Committee for Proprietary Medicinal Products Opinion Following an Article 31 Referral: Sibutramine. European Agency for the Evaluation of Medicinal Products Postauthorization Evaluation of Medicines for Human Use. December 2, 2002.
http://www.emea.eu.int/pdfs/human/referral/451402en.pdf

'Complications of Obesity', *WebMD* 2003.
http://www.medscape.com/viewarticle/457926_10

Craddock, D. 'Anorectic Drugs: Use in General Practice', *Drugs* 1976; 11(5): 378–93

Croft, H., *et al.* 'Effect on Body Weight of Bupropion Sustained-Release in Patients with Major Depression Treated for 52 Weeks', *Clinical Therapy* April 2002; 24(4): 662–72

Crook, William G. *The Yeast Connection: A Medical Breakthrough* (Vintage, 1986)

Crook, William G. and Cass, Hyla. *The Yeast Connection and Women's Health* (Professional Books, 2003)

Cummings, David E., *et al.* 'Plasma Ghrelin Levels After Diet-Induced Weight Loss or Gastric Bypass Surgery', *New England Journal of Medicine* May 23, 2002; 346(21): 1623–30

Dargent, J. 'Laparoscopic Adjustable Gastric Banding: Lessons from the First 500 Patients in a Single Institution', *Obesity Surgery* October 9, 1999; 5: 446–52

Diethylpropion. RXlist.com.
http://www.rxlist.com/frame/display.cgi?drug=TENUATE

Erasmus, Udo. *Fats That Heal, Fats That Kill* (Alive Books, 1999)

European Agency for the Evaluation of Medicinal Products. Press release. September 9, 1999.
http://www.emea.eu.int/pdfs/human/press/pr/232599en.pdf

European Journal of Clinical Nutrition 2002; 56: 740–47

Ezrin, Calvin. *Your Fat Can Make You Thin* (Contemporary Books, 2001)

Fat Cell Hormone Promotes Type 2 Diabetes. National Institutes of Health, National Institute of Diabetes and Digestive and Kidney Diseases. January 2001. http://www.niddk.nih.gov/welcome/releases/1-01.htm

Fen-Phen Online Information Resource. James F. Early, LLC, 2001.
http://www.fenphen-facts.com/overview_history.htm

Fife, Bruce. *The Healing Miracles of Coconut Oil* (Piccadilly Books, 2003)

Freudenrich, Craig C. 'How Fat Cells Work', *HowStuffWorks.com.*
http://home.howstuffworks.com/fat-cell.htm/printable

Fung, T. T., F. B. Hu, M. A. Pereira, *et al.* 'Whole-grain intake and the risk of type 2 diabetes: a prospective study in men', *American Journal of Clinical Nutrition* 2002; 76: 535–40

Gadde, Kishore. 'Long-Term Study Finds Antidepressants Effective for Weight Loss in Women', *DukeMed News Office* September 11, 2001

Galletti, Pierre-M., *et al.* 'Effect of Fluorine on the Thyroidal Iodine Metabolism in Hyperthyroidism', *Journal of Clinical Endocrinology* 1958; 18: 1102–10

Gate Pharmaceuticals. *Adipex-P (phentermine hydrochloride) Product Information.* November 2000. http://www.gatepharma.com/Adipex-P/adipexscript.pdf

Gittleman, Ann Louise. *Why Am I Always So Tired?* (HarperSanFrancisco, 1999)

———. *Eat Fat, Lose Weight* (Keats Publishing, 1999)

———. *The Fat Flush Plan* (McGraw-Hill, 2002)

———. *Guess What Came to Dinner? Parasites and Your Health* (Avery Penguin Putnam, 2001)

GlaxoSmithKline. *Wellbutrin SR (bupropion hydrochloride), Prescribing Information.* October 2002.
http://us.gsk.com/products/assets/us_wellbutrinSR.pdf

Glazer, G. 'Long-term Pharmacotherapy of Obesity 2000: A Review of Efficacy and Safety', *Archives of Internal Medicine* August 13–27, 2001; 161(15): 1814–24

Goglia, Philip L. *Turn Up the Heat: Unlock the Fat-Burning Power of Your Metabolism* (Viking, 2002)

Goode, Erica. 'The Heavy Cost of Chronic Stress', *New York Times*, December 17, 2002

Gortmaker, S. L., A. Must, J. M. Perrin, *et al.* 'Social and Economic Consequences of Overweight in Adolescence and Young Adulthood', *New England Journal of Medicine* 1993; 329: 1008

Grayson, Charlotte E. (ed). 'Insulin Resistance Syndrome', *WebMD Health*, November 2002

Grout, Pam. *Jumpstart Your Metabolism: How to Lose Weight by Changing the Way You Breathe* (Fireside, 1998)

Haines, Pamela S., *et al.* 'Weekend Eating in the United States Is Linked with Greater Energy, Fat and Alcohol Intake', *Obesity Research* 2003; 11: 945–49

Hanks, Bart and Ric Rooney. *The Physique Transformation Program.* http://www.physiquetransformation.com

Harrison, Lewis. *Master Your Metabolism* (Sourcebooks, Inc., 2003)

Hayashi T., *et al.* 'Ellagitannins from Lagerstroemia speciosa as Activators of Glucose Transport in Fat Cells', *Planta Medica* 2002; 68(2): 173–75

Heavin, Gary. *Curves: Permanent Results Without Permanent Dieting* (G. P. Putnam's Sons, 2003)

Indications and Side-Effects. Presentations at American Epilepsy Society 56th Annual Meeting, December 2002

Insulin Resistance and Pre-Diabetes. National Institutes of Health, National Institute of Diabetes and Digestive and Kidney Diseases, National Diabetes Information Clearinghouse. May 2003. http://www.idd.nih.gov/health/diabetes/pubs/insulinres/index.htm

'Insulin Resistance Syndrome', American Academy of Family Physicians. *American Family Physician* March 15, 2001

Jahnke, Roger O. 'Oxygen Metabolism', *HealthWorld.* http://www.healthy.net/asp/templates/article.asp?PageType=Article&ID=991

Jonsson, S., B. Hedblad, G. Engstrom, *et al.* 'Influence of Obesity on Cardiovascular Risk: Twenty-Three-Year Follow-up of 22,025 Men from an Urban Swedish Population', *International Journal of Obesity Related Metabolic Disorders* 2002; 26: 1046

Judy, W. V., *et al.* 'Antidiabetic Activity of a Standardized Extract (Glucosol) from *Lagerstroemia speciosa* Leaves in Type II Diabetics. A Dose-Dependence Study', *Journal of Ethnopharmacology* July 2003; 87(1): 115–17

Kakuda, T., I. Sakane, T. Takihara, Y. Ozaki, H. Takeuchi and M. Kuroyanagi. 'Hypoglycemic Effect of Extracts from *Lagerstroemia speciosa L.* Leaves in Genetically Diabetic KK-AY Mice', *Bioscience. Biotechnology and Biochemistry* February 1996; 60(2): 204–208

Kalfarentzos, F., *et al.* 'Weight Loss Following Vertical Banded Gastroplasty: Intermediate Results of a Prospective Study', *Obesity Surgery* June 2001; 11(3): 265–70

Kolata, Gina. 'The Fat Epidemic/New Clues from the Lab/How the Body Knows When to Gain or Lose', *New York Times* Science Section, October 17, 2000

Krotkiewski, M. 'Thyroid Hormones in the Pathogenesis and Treatment of Obesity', *European Journal of Pharmacology* April 12, 2002; 440(2–3): 85–98

Lakka, H. M., D. E. Laaksonen, T. A., Lakka, *et al.* 'The Metabolic Syndrome and Cardiovascular Disease Mortality in Middle-aged Men', *Journal of the American Medical Association* 2002; 288: 2709

Langer, Stephen and James F. Scheer. *Solved: The Riddle of Illness* (Healing Arts Press, 1989)

Layton, Julia. 'How Calories Work', *HowStuffWorks.com.* http://home.howstuffworks.com/calorie.htm/printable

Leeds, A. R. 'Glycemic Index and Heart Disease', *American Journal of Clinical Nutrition* 2002; 76: 286S–289S

Lejeune, Manuela. 'Additional Protein Intake Limits Weight Gain After Weight Loss in Humans. Abstract t4: 02', *Proceedings of the European Congress of Obesity*, Helsinki, Finland, June, 2003

Linquette, A. and P. Fossati. 'Hunger Control with Benzphetamine Hydrochloride in the Treatment of Obesity', *Lille Medical*, April 1971; 16(suppl 2): 620–24

Liu, F., J. Kim, Y. Li, X. Liu, J. Li and X. Chen. 'An Extract of Lagerstroemia speciosa L. Has Insulin-like Glucose Uptake-Stimulatory and Adipocyte Differentiation-Inhibitory Activities in 3T3-L1 Cells', *Journal of Nutrition* September 2001; 131(9): 2242–47

Liu, S., W. C. Willett, M. J. Stampfer, F. B. Hu, *et al.* 'A Prospective Study of Dietary Glycemic Load, Carbohydrate Intake and Risk of Coronary Heart Disease in US Women', *American Journal of Clinical Nutrition* 2000; 71: 1455–61

MacGregor, Alex (ed). *The Story of Surgery for Obesity*, American Society of Bariatric Surgeons (ASBS), 2002 Amendment

Manson, J. E., W. C. Willett, M. J. Stampfer, *et al.* 'Body Weight and Mortality Among Women', *New England Journal of Medicine* 1995; 333: 677. *Medscape*

Mason, E. E. 'Vertical Banded Gastroplasty for Obesity', *Archives of Surgery* May 1982; 117(5): 701–6

———. 'Why the Operation I Prefer Is Vertical Banded Gastroplasty', *Obesity Surgery* June 1991; 1(2): 181–83

Mason, E. E. and C. Ito. 'Gastric Bypass in Obesity', *Surgical Clinics of North America* December 1967; 47(6): 1345–51

Mason, E. E., *et al.* 'Gastric Bypass for Obesity After Ten Years' Experience', *International Journal of Obesity* 1978; 2(2): 197–206

Mazansky, H. 'A Review of Obesity and Its Management in 263 Cases', *South African Medical Journal* November 8, 1975; 49(47): 1955–62

'Medical Encyclopedia: Obesity', *MEDLINEplus.* May 17, 2002. http://www.nlm.nih.gov/medlineplus/ency/article/003101.htm#Definition

Meigs, J. B. 'The Metabolic Syndrome', *British Medical Journal* 2003; 327: 61–62

Mellin, Laurel. *The Solution: 6 Winning Ways to Permanent Weight Loss* (Regan Books, 1997)

Mercola, Joseph and Alison Rose Levy. *The No-Grain Diet: Conquer Carbohydrate Addiction and Stay Slim for Life* (E. P. Dutton, 2003)

'Mesotherapy FAQ', *Mesotherapie & Estetik.* http://mesoestetik.com/faq.html

'Mesotherapy Overview', Health Plus web. *Directory of Alternative Medicine.* http://www.healthplusweb.com/alt_directory/mesotherapy.html

Michaud, Ellen. 'Healing with Your Sixth Sense', *Prevention*, May 2003

Miller, Peter M. *The Hilton Head Metabolism Diet* (Warner Books, 1983)

Mogul, Harriette, *et al. The Endocrinopathy of Obesity: Correlate, Consequence or Cause?* Abstracts, 84th annual meeting of the Endocrine Society, June 2002

Mokdad, A. H., E. S. Ford, B. A. Bowman, *et al.* 'Prevalence of Obesity, Diabetes and Obesity-Related Health Risk Factors, 2001', *Journal of the American Medical Association* 2003; 289: 76

Muller, F. O., *et al.* 'Availability of Phendimetrazine from Sustained and Non-Sustained Action Formula', *South African Medical Journal* February 1, 1975; 49(5): 135–39

Murakami, C., K. Myoga, R. Kasai, K. Ohtani, T. Kurokawa, S. Ishibashi, F. Dayrit, W. G. Padolina and K. Yamasaki. 'Screening of Plant Constituents for Effect on Glucose Transport Activity in Ehrlich Ascites Tumour Cells', *Chemical and Pharmaceutical Bulletin* (Tokyo), December 1993; 41(12): 2129–31

Must, A., J. Spadano, E. H. Coakley, *et al.* 'The Disease Burden Associated with Overweight and Obesity', *Journal of the American Medical Association* 1999; 282: 1523

O'Brien, P. E., *et al.* 'Prospective Study of a Laparoscopically Placed, Adjustablic Gastric Band in the Treatment of Morbid Obesity', *British Journal of Surgery* January 1999; 86(1): 113–118

'One-Year Prophylactic Treatment of Euthyroid Hashimoto's Thyroiditis Patients with Levothyroxine: Is There a Benefit?', *Thyroid* March 2001; 11(3): 249–55

Orlistat. RXList.com. http://www.rxlist.com/frame/display.cgi?drug=Xenical

Osono, Y., N. Hirose, K. Nakajima and Y. Hata. Y. 'The Effects of Pantethine on Fatty Liver and Fat Distribution', *Journal of Atherosclerosis and Thrombosis* 2000; 7(1): 55–58

Overweight and Obesity, Defining Overweight and Obesity. Centers for Disease Control and Prevention, National Center for Chronic Disease Prevention and Health Promotion, Division of Nutrition and Physical Activity. April 22, 2003.
http://www.cdc.gov/nccdphp/dnpa/obesity/defining.htm

Palkhivala, Alison. 'New Hormone Might Explain Link Between Diabetes and Obesity', *WebMD Health* January 17, 2001

Parsons, W. B., Jr. 'Controlled-Release Diethylpropion Hydrochloride Used in a Program for Weight Reduction', *Clinical Therapy* 1981; 3(5): 329–35

Peppard, P. E., T. Young, M. Palta, *et al.* 'Longitudinal Study of Moderate Weight Change and Sleep-Disordered Breathing', *Journal of the American Medical Association* 2000; 284: 3015

Perrone, Tony. *Dr Tony Perrone's Body Fat Breakthru* (Regan Books, 1999)

Pharmacia & Upjohn Company. *Didrex (benzphetamine hydrochloride) Product Information*. April 2002.
   http://www.pfizer.com/download/uspi_didrex.pdf

Phendimetrazine Information. Eon Labs. June 16, 1999.
   http://www.phendimetrazine.org/phendimetrazine-information.htm

Phendimetrazine. RXlist.com.
   http://www.rxlist.com/frame/display.cgi?drug=BONTRIL

Phentermine. RXlist.com.
   http://www.rxlist.com/frame/display.cgi?drug=ADIPEX

Pijl, *et al.* 'Food Choice in Hyperthyroidism: Potential Influence of the Autonomic Nervous System and Brain Serotonin Precursor Availability', *Journal of Clinical Endocrinology and Metabolism* 2001; 86(12): 5848–53

Pi-Sunyer, F. X. 'Medical Hazards of Obesity', *Annals of Internal Medicine* 1993; 19: 655

Plauchu, M., *et al.* 'Trial of Benzphetamine in Treatment of Obesity', *Lyon Medical* September 14, 1969; 222(32): 317–21

Proceedings of the National Academy of Sciences Early Edition 2002; 10.1073/pnas.132128899

Proceedings of the National Academy of Sciences 2003; 10.1073/pnas.0636646100

Product Review: Weight Loss, Slimming and Diabetes-Management Supplements (Chromium, CLA and Pyruvate) Consumerlab.com

Psychosomatic Medicine 2002; 64: 593–603

Purnell, M. D. and Q. Jonathan. 'What's New in Medicine: Obesity', *WebMD Scientific American® Medicine* 2003.
   http://www.medscape.com/viewarticle/456351

Report of the Dietary Guidelines Advisory Committee on the Dietary Guidelines for Americans, 2000: 3

Richards, Byron. *Mastering Leptin* (Wellness Resources, 2003)

Rimm, E. B., M. J. Stampfer, E. Giovannucci, *et al.* 'Body Size and Fat Distribution as Predictors of Coronary Heart Disease Among Middle-aged and Older US Men', *American Journal of Epidemiology* 1995; 141: 1117

Roche Laboratories Inc. *Xenical (Orlistat) Capsules, Product Information*. September 2000. http://www.rocheusa.com/products/xenical/pi.html

Rooney, Ric and Bart Hanks. *Secrets of a Professional Dieter*. Ebook. http://www.physiquetransformation.com

Rosch, Paul J. 'Stress and Why All Obesity Is Not Created Equal', *Red Flags Daily Online Magazine*, April 14, 2003. http://www.redflagsdaily.com

Ross, Julia. *The Diet Cure* (Viking Penguin, 1999)

Rubenstein R. 'Laparoscopic Adjustable Gastric Banding at a U.S. Center with Up to 3-Year Follow-up', *Obesity Surgery* 2002; 12: 380–4

St-Onge, M. P., 'Physiological Effects of Medium-Chain Triglycerides: Potential Agents in the Prevention of Obesity', *Journal of Nutrition* March 2002; 132(3): 329–32

Samaha, Frederick, *et al.* 'A Low-Carbohydrate as Compared with a Low-Fat Diet in Severe Obesity', *New England Journal of Medicine* May 22, 2003; 348: 2074–81

Sanalkumar, Nishanth, *et al. Prevalence and Potential Implications of Undetected Thyroid Abnormalities in a Population of Obese Patients*, Abstracts, 84th annual meeting of the Endocrine Society, June 2002

Sankar, Raman. 'Anticonvulsants: Newest Clinical Trials Focus on Potential', American Epilepsy Society 56th Annual Meeting, December 2002. http://www.medscape.com/viewprogram/2253

Savard, Marie. *How to Save Your Own Life: The Savard System for Managing – and Controlling – Your Health Care* (Warner Books, 2000)
———. *The Savard Health Record: A Six-Step System for Managing Your Health Care* (Time Life, 2000)

Scopinaro, N., *et al.* 'Biliopancreatic Diversion for Obesity at Eighteen Years', *Surgery* March 1996; 119(3): 261–68

Seeley, Rod R., Trent D. Stephens and Philip Tate. *Anatomy and Physiology* (St Louis, MO: Time Mirror/Mosby College Publishing, 1989)

Shames, Richard and Karilee Halo Shames. *Thyroid Power: Ten Steps to Total Health* (Harper Resource, 2001)

Sibutramine. RXlist.com. http://www.rxlist.com/frame/display.cgi?drug=Meridia

Simontacchi, Carol. *Your Fat Is Not Your Fault* (Penguin Putnam Inc., 1998)

Sjorstrom, Lars, *et al.* 'Randomized Placebo-Controlled Trial of Orlistat for Weight Loss and Prevention of Weight Gain in Obese Patients', *Lancet* July 18, 1998; 352(9123): 167–73. http://www.thelancet.com/search/search.isa

Spiegel, K., R. Leproult and E. Van Cauter. 'Impact of sleep debt on metabolic and endocrine function', *Lancet* 1999; 354: 1435–39

Strauss, R. S. 'Childhood Obesity and Self-Esteem', *Pediatrics* 2000; 105: e15

Studies Show Xenical (Orlistat) Helps Patients with Type 2 Diabetes Lose Weight and Attain Improved Control of Their Diabetes with Less Anti-Diabetic Medications. Roche Laboratories Inc., November 6, 2000. http://www.rocheusa.com/news room/current/2000/pr2000110601.html

Suzuki, Y., T. Unno, M. Ushitani, K. Hayashi and T. Kakuda. 'Antiobesity Activity of Extracts from *Lagerstroemia speciosa L.* Leaves on Female KK-Ay Mice', *Journal of Nutritional Science and Vitaminology* (Tokyo), December 1999; 45(6): 791–95

Taubes, Gary. 'What If It's All Been a Big Fat Lie?', *New York Times,* July 2, 2002

Teitelbaum, Jacob. *From Fatigued to Fantastic* (Avery Penguin Putnam, 2001)

Telles, S., R. Nagarathna and H. R. Nagendra. 'Breathing Through a Particular Nostril Can Alter Metabolism and Autonomic Activities', *Indian J. Physiol. Pharmacol* April 1994; 38(2): 133

Topiramate. RXlist.com. www.rxlist.com/frame/display.cgi?drug opamax

U.S. Food and Drug Administration. Letter to Eon Labs (manufacturer of phendimetazine) about updating the product information for the drug. November 3, 1998. http://www.fda.gov/cder/ogd/rld/18074s28.pdf

Valle-Jones, J. C., *et al.* 'A Comparative Study of Phentermine and Diethylpropion in the Treatment of Obese Patients in General Practices', *Pharmatherapeutica* 1983; 3(5): 300–4

Van Cauter, E., R. Leproult and L. Plat. 'Age-Related Changes in Slow Wave Sleep and REM Sleep and Relationship with Growth Hormone and Cortisol Levels in Healthy Men', *Journal of the American Medical Association* 2000; 284: 861–68

Vitamin C May Help 'Juice Up' Metabolism in Older Adults, Offsetting Weight Gain. University of Colorado at Boulder press release. April, 2002

Weintraub, M., *et al.* 'A Double-Blind Clinical Trial in Weight Control: Use of Fenfluramine and Phentermine Alone and in Combination', *Archives of Internal Medicine* June 1984; 144(6): 1143–48

Where's the Fat?
http://www.thedoctorwillseeyounow.com/articles/nutrition/fatdistribut
ion_1/fat_distribution_appendix.shtml

Willett, W. J. Manson and S. Liu. 'Glycemic Index, Glycemic Load and
Risk of Type 2 Diabetes', *American Journal of Clinical Nutrition*
2002; 76(suppl.)274S–280S

Wittgrove, C. and G. W. Clark. 'Laparoscopic Gastric Bypass, Roux-en-Y-
500 Patients. Technique and Results with 3–60 Month Follow-up',
Obesity Surgery 2000; 10: 233–39

Wolcott, William Linz and Trish Fahey. *The Metabolic Typing Diet:
Customize Your Diet to Your Own Unique Body Chemistry* (Broadway
Books, 2002)

Wolever, T. M. and C. Mehling. 'High-Carbohydrate-Low-Glycaemic
Index Dietary Advice Improves Glucose Disposition Index in Subjects
with Impaired Glucose Tolerance', *British Journal of Nutrition* 2002;
87: 477–87

Wolf, A. M. and G. A. Colditz. 'Current Estimates of the Economic Cost of
Obesity in the United States', *Obesity Research* 1998; 6: 97

Index